# Post-Traumatic Stress Disorder

# Post-Traumatic Stress Disorder

Stanley Krippner, PhD,
Daniel B. Pitchford, PhD, and
Jeannine Davies, PhD

Biographies of Disease
*Julie K. Silver, M.D., Series Editor*

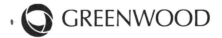

AN IMPRINT OF ABC-CLIO, LLC
Santa Barbara, California • Denver, Colorado • Oxford, England

**Library of Congress Cataloging-in-Publication Data**

Krippner, Stanley, 1932–
    Post-traumatic stress disorder / Stanley Krippner, Daniel B. Pitchford, and Jeannine Davies.
        p. cm. — (Biographies of disease)
    Includes bibliographical references and index.
    ISBN 978–0–313–38668–8 (hardback) — ISBN 978–0–313–38669–5 (ebook)
1. Post-traumatic stress disorder. 2. Post-traumatic stress disorder—Physiological aspects. 3. Post-traumatic stress disorder—Treatment. I. Pitchford, Daniel. II. Davies, Jeannine. III. Title.
RC552.P67K75   2012
616.85′21—dc23          2011045335

ISBN: 978–0–313–38668–8
EISBN: 978–0–313–38669–5

16  15  14  13  12      1  2  3  4  5

This book is also available on the World Wide Web as an eBook.
Visit www.abc-clio.com for details.

Greenwood
An Imprint of ABC-CLIO, LLC

ABC-CLIO, LLC
130 Cremona Drive, P.O. Box 1911
Santa Barbara, California 93116-1911

This book is printed on acid-free paper ∞

Manufactured in the United States of America

Portions of this book were originally published in Daryl S. Paulson and Stanley Krippner, *Haunted by Combat: Understanding PTSD in War Veterans Including Women, Reservists, and Those Coming Back from Iraq.* © 2007 by Daryl S. Paulson and Stanley Krippner. Reproduced with permission of ABC-CLIO, LLC, Santa Barbara, CA.

*The authors dedicate this book to those women and men, girls and boys, who have survived trauma, and to the health care providers, significant others, and support groups who have assisted them in their struggle.*

# Contents

# Series Foreword

E very disease has a story to tell: about how it started long ago and began to disable or even take the lives of its innocent victims, about the way it hurts us, and about how we are trying to stop it. In this Biographies of Disease series, the authors tell the stories of the diseases that we have come to know and dread.

The stories of these diseases have all of the components that make for great literature. There is incredible drama played out in real-life scenes from the past, present, and future. You'll read about how men and women of science stumbled trying to save the lives of those they aimed to protect. Turn the pages and you'll also learn about the amazing success of those who fought for health and won, often saving thousands of lives in the process.

If you don't want to be a health professional or research scientist now, when you finish this book you may think differently. The men and women in this book are heroes who often risked their own lives to save or improve ours. This is the biography of a disease, but it is also the story of real people who made incredible sacrifices to stop it in its tracks.

Julie K. Silver, M.D.
Assistant Professor, Harvard Medical School
Department of Physical Medicine and Rehabilitation

# Acknowledgments

T he authors acknowledge the editorial assistance they received in the preparation of this book from Rosemary Coffey, Leslie Allan Combs, Steven M. Hart, and Christopher Sadowski, as well as the financial support from the Saybrook University Chair for the Study of Consciousness, and a special contribution from the Leir Family Trust.

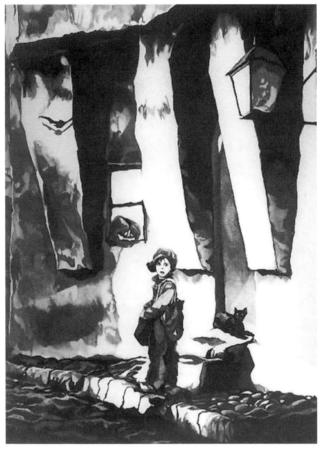

Andy Heck (Reproduced from the original art of Dierdre Luzwick.)

# Trauma: An Introduction

Margaret lived a life full of purpose and determination that had helped her to fulfill her life-long dreams. She was supported in pursuing these life goals by her husband of over 20 years. Both Margaret and her husband were committed to their marriage and to supporting each other throughout life.

But six months before their 26th wedding anniversary, Margaret's life was suddenly shattered when her husband was killed in a tragic industrial accident. Margaret found herself feeling numb and without a sense of direction in her life. In the days and months that followed the funeral, Margaret stopped working and seeing friends, preferring instead to stay in her home. Eventually, Margaret did not even attend to the simplest tasks of personal hygiene, wearing a housecoat that she rarely changed. In addition, Margaret's sudden confrontation with the reality of death invaded her outlook on life and unveiled the fact that all living things must come to an end.

Many people of all ages have either witnessed or personally endured a stressful life event or circumstance such as the loss of a relationship, the death of a family member or friend, a natural disaster, sexual or emotional abuse, family violence, or war. How people encounter and internalize such events, as well as how those circumstances are viewed by the culture in which they live, affect how these events will impact their lives.

More often than not, life events cannot be predicted, nor are circumstances always consistent with people's desires or their wish for control. Yet it is precisely this unpredictability that yields a consistent effect, influencing and shaping people's development, beliefs, and overall life experiences. Change is an undeniable factor of existence. From the impact of earthquakes, floods, hurricanes, and other natural disasters to the role that a simple misunderstanding can play in disrupting a romantic relationship, the processes of change are inevitably at work. However, it is through understanding and accepting the nature of change and its pervasive influence upon the stressful events of everyday life (such as sickness, divorce, aging, unemployment, or loss) that people have the opportunity to develop greater resiliency and nurture the capacity to live a richer life. Not surprisingly, people's encounter with trauma is no exception.

The word "trauma," which originated in the late 17th century, is derived from a Greek word for "wound." In the most general sense, a wound implies that an injury has occurred. Sometimes, this injury may be physical, and at other times it may be psychological. Although psychological wounding—an injury to the psyche due to a traumatizing event—can occur along with a physical wound, bodily harm is not necessary for an emotional reaction to develop. The intensity (minor or major) of wounding that occurs is directly connected to how an individual experiences, thinks, and feels about a traumatizing encounter, activity, or occurrence.

How people experience their wounding brought on by a traumatizing event is strongly related to their personal temperament, personal history (especially any prior traumas), context (the setting or environment), and the subjective impact of the event—in other words, how they attribute meaning to what has happened. For example, if parents decide to divorce, their behavior regarding that decision can strongly impact how the divorce is perceived and experienced by their child or children. Some children blame themselves for their parents' decision to divorce, while others feel neglected and betrayed by the disruption of the family unit. However, if parents are respectful and honest about the choices being made, and take responsibility for behavior around each other and with their children, the stress on the children will be reduced. On the other hand, if parents are angry, bitter, and demeaning of each other, their children's already stressful life experience will be augmented by the harmful nature of the parents' behavior. This conduct may increase the severity of the wound inflicted on the children, leaving long-lasting scars on their vulnerable psyches.

It is in this way that psychological wounds, often less visible to the naked eye than physical wounds, are revealed both in relation to the particular nature of the traumatizing event and the beliefs and attitudes of the person who has been impacted. Many centuries ago, the Greek philosopher Epictetus wrote, "It is not what happens to you, but how you react to it that is important" (White, 1983, p. 11). Events might shape one's life, but the meanings that an individual attaches to those events will be even more influential. Recognizing the difference between an "event" and an "experience" is crucial to the understanding of trauma.

The effects of trauma upon the individual can manifest in varied ways. For some, trauma can leave emotional scars that impact all future relationships. For example, if a person has been raped, he or she may no longer be able or willing to trust people of the perpetrator's gender, age, or ethnic group. In other types of abuse, trauma may manifest through discomfort and stress that, when not recognized accurately, can take on bizarre forms of expression such as avoidance of social gatherings, sudden bursts of profanity, or simmering anger and resentment.

An example would be an act of violence within an intimate relationship. The behavior of the abuser in the relationship can have such a severe effect on the partner that he or she may be consumed with overwhelming suspicion, paranoia, and even hallucinations. If the context or story of that individual's life is not understood, he or she may easily be misdiagnosed as schizophrenic, for example, rather than as a person who has been traumatized.

Understanding the culture, the subcultures, and the social contexts in which people live is crucial in appreciating the full spectrum of experiences that may be impacting and shaping their lives. An event that traumatizes people in one culture may be shrugged off as a daily occurrence in another one. Piercing the skin during a coming-of-age ritual may be experienced as a mark of maturity in a tribal society, but the same intervention could be traumatizing to a person raised in a Western culture, one who lacks the context and meaning to reduce the pain and appreciate the privilege of this act.

## COMPLEXITY OF TRAUMA

The ways in which trauma can impact individuals and groups are both dramatic and dynamic. This can be illustrated by imagining a tragic shooting at a school that involves both students and teachers. In the event of such a shooting, the student or teacher who is physically injured will usually be more severely affected emotionally than the student or teacher who witnesses the shooting. Yet those witnesses are likely to be more impacted emotionally than students who were in another part of the school when the violence occurred.

At the same time, the degree of trauma that manifests is linked not only to the school setting, but also to the life history and home environment of both students and teachers. An exchange student from a turbulent part of the world, where violence is a daily affair may assimilate the shooting episode more quickly than a student whose home environment has been placid and free from violence. However, it is important to note that while the latter student is typically more susceptible to developing traumatic stress, this is not always the case. Some people simply lack the empathy to put themselves in the place of those individuals who are injured in an attack, even one that they personally witness.

Those people who watched the World Trade Center towers fall to the ground on September 11, 2001, may recall the televised or filmed images of the airplanes crashing into the skyscrapers. Although it may manifest itself in subtle ways, this vicarious form of exposure can be traumatic to some degree. For this reason, some people exposed to a disaster, even if only through graphic media, are susceptible to the psychological impact of trauma. In addition to how people respond individually to trauma, how they respond to each other affects the overall impact. An example of the latter was apparent in the case of U.S. combat soldiers who served in Vietnam. When they returned home from their service, many were accosted and verbally attacked for the role that they played in that conflict, a hostile reception that had many negative effects upon some veterans' ability to readjust to civilian life. Similar unsympathetic receptions did not characterize the homecoming of combat veterans who served in Iraq and Afghanistan, even though there was considerable civilian opposition to those conflicts.

On the other hand, a person living in an extended family may be offered considerably more sympathy and compassion than if he or she lives alone or with one or two others. This contrasts with the situation of people living in cultures that take pride in restraining emotions and "keeping a stiff upper lip." In those cases, they may have more difficulty coping with the trauma than those living in a culture where feelings are expressed openly and where the trauma survivor can "let it all hang out."

You will notice that we are using the term "trauma survivor" instead of "trauma victim" or "trauma sufferer." Our aim throughout this book is to focus on ways in which people who have undergone traumatic experiences cannot only recover, but thrive, developing "post-traumatic strengths" along the way. To "victimize" people who have undergone trauma is to emphasize the negative aspects of their experience; such terminology may even *retraumatize* individuals, and derail their recovery.

You will also notice that we speak of *traumatizing events* and *traumatic experiences*. A catastrophic event such as a car crash is *potentially traumatizing* to the occupants of that automobile. Some will assimilate the experience and bounce back easily. For others, that event will be *traumatizing* and will become a *traumatic experience*. The words used when discussing trauma need to be carefully chosen to honor the individual differences of individuals who have been subjected to forms of stress so intense that they are, indeed, potentially traumatizing.

## THE TRAUMA RESPONSE

In other words, it is important to remember that it is not the event that determines whether something is traumatizing, but the individual's *experience* of the event. Several factors may *predispose* one individual to being more susceptible to emotional and psychological stress than another. These include previous traumas such as living in unstable or unsafe environments, separation from a parent, serious illness, intrusive medical procedures, domestic violence, emotional neglect, bullying, and sexual, physical, or verbal abuse. These predisposing factors could also include grieving a recent loss or experiencing a significant level of stress at the time of the traumatizing event. Although these factors may predispose an individual to be more vulnerable to trauma, it is not entirely predictable how a given person will react to a particular circumstance. People are volatile, especially when emotional issues are at play. For people who are used to being in control of their emotions, it may be surprising—and even embarrassing—for them to discover that being injured in sports, failing an exam, or having a relationship fall apart can be extremely debilitating.

As noted above, the distinguishing characteristic of what makes an event traumatizing is how the event is perceived and experienced. For example, for one person, public speaking might be an exhilarating challenge, while for another it might be terrifying and stressful. If an event is perceived as overwhelmingly stressful, one's ability to easily integrate that experience becomes less likely and the odds of it leading to a traumatic experience may increase.

The American Psychological Association's *Dictionary of Psychology* defines "trauma" as an occurrence "in which a person witnesses or experiences a threat to his or her own life or physical safety or that of others and experiences fear, terror, or helplessness. . . . [Such occurrences] challenge an individual's view of the world as a just, safe, and predictable place" (VandenBos, 2006, p. 955). Events that might be experienced as traumatic include transportation collisions, toxic accidents, natural disasters, human-made disasters, forced incarceration, assault, or witnessing an assault. Less obvious examples of traumatizing events could include sports injuries, invasive surgery, the sudden death of a loved one, hearing a graphic account about violence, the breakup of a significant relationship, a humiliating or deeply disappointing experience, or being informed about a loved one's life-threatening illness or disabling condition. We have cited some of these circumstances before, but some repetition will help you, the reader, become aware of the wide range of potentially traumatizing events.

Traumatic stress is a normal response to an extreme event, one that is outside a person's ordinary life experiences. The intensity of this response triggers the creation of emotional memories linked with the stressful event, which then become stored within the brain and body. In general, the more direct the exposure to the traumatic event, the higher the risk for emotional harm. The risk of susceptibility to becoming traumatized and the onset of subsequent disorders are based on three elements: (1) The traumatizing occurrence is unexpected; (2) The person is not prepared for the experience; and (3) In most cases, nothing could have been done to prevent the experience from happening (Herman, 1997; Lapin, 1997).

## RESPONDING TO TRAUMA

An individual's perception and experience of the traumatizing event will determine where the response falls on the trauma spectrum. Stress can be psychological, physiological, or both, and can affect almost every bodily system. Variations in stress can range from mild to severe; in the latter instance, the so-called "general adaptation syndrome," the consequences of intense stress, can impair a person's functioning so badly that his or her quality of life is significantly reduced. Stress can evoke sweating, palpitations, shortness of breath, a dry mouth, negative moods, and other manifestations.

People typically experience the same event in different ways. One example that highlights this principle can be seen through the horror of war combat. Two soldiers may endure the same exposure to the trauma of being shot at while shooting at an enemy. Yet, it is possible that only one of them may go on to develop overwhelming stress that leads to a diagnosis of post-traumatic stress disorder (PTSD). If the soldier is impacted by other life traumas (for example, abuse, loss, accusations), his or her susceptibility to developing serious symptoms may be greater (Pitchford, 2009).

While no one knows exactly what factors (including biological predispositions or a low capacity for resilience) are involved in a predisposition to PTSD, there are various causal factors that contribute to the disorder. For example, school violence is viewed as a human-made disaster, whereas earthquakes are considered natural disasters. The type of disaster itself may determine the level of PTSD a person experiences, depending upon how the survivor's sense of invulnerability to harm is challenged. Also, it is important to note that young adults commonly display a sense of imperviousness to being wounded and a heightened sense of transcendent immunity to life events. Both of these perspectives make susceptibility to a trauma's impact even greater (Paulson & Krippner, 2007). When a young person's notion of invulnerability is challenged, his or her entire worldview might be shaken.

In the case of a natural disaster, one's locus of control (the potential ability to take charge of an event) may be basically external in nature. For example, the Indian Ocean tsunami in 2004 could not have been prevented. As a result of there being no early warning systems in place to detect tsunamis in the Indian Ocean (unlike in the Pacific Ocean), people who lived along the coastal areas were given no notice. Following the disaster, further uncertainty was experienced as some people thought it would be safe to continue living where the disaster occurred, while others believed that moving away would be advisable until a warning system was implemented. Here again, one can see two different personal perspectives at work. Those survivors who saw the rationale for both of these scenarios could have felt caught in the middle of a personal conflict. Two *personal myths* were at play, and each one made a certain amount of sense, leading to a *mythological conflict*, a rupture in one's worldview.

Due to the uniqueness of each situation that involves trauma, it is especially important to understand the type of trauma that has occurred and the variety of reactions to it. By doing so, caregivers may be able to choose the most effective methods of intervening (for example, establishing survivor support groups, providing relief aid for displacement caused by the tsunami, providing quick burial of the dead to prevent disease, while concurrently allowing for a period of mourning with the accompanying cultural bereavement ceremonies).

While each person responds to stressful events uniquely, there are common emotional and physical symptoms that can accompany a trauma and may assist a mental health provider to make a formal diagnosis of PTSD. These symptoms may last for days, weeks, or even months, and may include:

- Shock, denial, or disbelief
- Anger, irritability, or mood swings
- Guilt, shame, or self-blame
- Feelings of sadness or hopelessness
- Confusion, with difficulty concentrating
- Anxiety and fear
- Withdrawal from others
- Feelings of disconnectedness or numbness

Common physical symptoms accompanying a traumatic experience include:

- Insomnia or nightmares
- Being startled easily
- A racing heartbeat
- Aches and pains
- Fatigue
- Edginess and agitation
- Muscle tension

## SUMMARY

The emotional and physical symptoms that can arise from and reflect trauma are by no means predictors of a disorder. Rather, they can be understood as a barometer of something occurring within an individual where the emotional complexity that is being encountered is overriding the ability to easily and rapidly integrate the experience. To some extent, these symptoms can be seen as a sane response to an insane world (Laing, 1965). It is in this way that we might view the expression of the symptoms listed above as a normal response to a stressful life event, evoked by an unfamiliar terrain of experience that is difficult to assimilate. Viewing trauma from this mindset allows both those who are observing the symptoms and those who are experiencing them to bring compassion and understanding to what is occurring. In so doing, the harmful effects that can follow from the stigma of "something being wrong" are reduced.

As this chapter has revealed, the nature of trauma is dramatic and dynamic, and responses to it vary. The factors that contribute to its onset arise both from the individual and from that person's cultural context. As a result, it is important to understand the framework from which mental health practitioners operate when someone manifests some or most of these symptoms. Among most Western psychotherapists, that framework will include the possible diagnosis of post-traumatic stress disorder, or PTSD.

# 2

# Recognizing PTSD

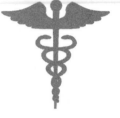

everal times a week, Betty wakes up following a terrifying nightmare. In some of these frightening dreams, her father is whipping her with a belt. Betty's mother is standing by helplessly, not doing anything to stop the abuse. In other nightmares, Betty's mother is being beaten and Betty is the help-less one. The interpretation of these dreams does not require a psychoanalyst. When Betty was a girl, her father would often come home intoxicated from a night at the bar. Betty would try to hide, but her father would find her, take off his belt, and start whipping her. One time Betty's mother threatened to call the police, but Betty's father said to her, "If you pick up that telephone, I will kill Betty." When Betty tried to stop her mother from being beaten, she was told the same thing: "If you put yourself between me and your mother, I will kill you both." When Betty was seven, her father was shot to death during a tavern brawl. Betty and her mother thought that their suffering had ended, but it simply took another form. Twenty years later, Betty was still having nightmares in which the abuse was inflicted again. Betty's mother also suffered from nightmares as well as from a host of other symptoms of PTSD.

People never know what any given moment might bring. The only constant in life is change, and there is no escaping it. One's biological, psychological, and spiritual being changes daily, through what is consumed, what is communi-cated, what is perceived, where one lives, and especially through how one cares (or does not care) for oneself. Oftentimes, changes can evoke stressful reactions (such as anger, anxiety, or despondence), as people attempt to maneuver through their daily encounters and find some sense of equilibrium. If these encounters become too stressful for people to manage easily, their body and psyche will react as best they can to counter the internal and external stressors that impact them. If these stressors are too overwhelming, however, stress reactions can leave people feeling helpless, depressed, or anxious.

Not everyone who endures such episodes becomes traumatized. A catastrophic event, such as seeing a friend swept out to sea and drowned, may be gradually assimilated by one person, but not by another. The friend's death is not traumatizing for the first person, but becomes a traumatic experience for the second one. For the latter, and for others who are susceptible, their attitudes and behaviors makes them eligible for a psychiatric diagnosis such as "acute stress disorder" or, in more severe cases, "post-traumatic stress disorder" (PTSD). Mild stress is at one end of the spectrum, acute stress disorder falls in the middle, and various types of PTSD represent the extreme end. The number of symptoms, the severity of symptoms, and the length that the symptoms persist determine where someone falls on the trauma spectrum.

The term "post-traumatic stress disorder" is relatively new. It first appeared in 1980, in the American Psychiatric Association's *Diagnostic and Statistical Manual of Mental Disorders* (*DSM*, 3rd and 4th editions, 1980 and 1994) and in 1977, in the World Health Organization's *International Statistical Classification of Diseases and Related Health Problems* (*ICD*, 9th and 10th editions, 1977 and 1992). While these classification systems are used throughout the world, they reflect Western cultural beliefs about human nature. Thus, it is necessary to consider cultural implications when a mental health practitioner makes a formal diagnosis. This topic will be discussed more thoroughly in Chapter 3.

In the United States, the diagnosis of PTSD was developed in the late 1970s when a sizable number of veterans returning home from the Vietnam Conflict behaved in ways that appeared to be associated with high levels of psychological distress. Because the emotional problems faced by those who had served in Vietnam were major motivators for PTSD to receive recognition as a disorder, many people associate PTSD with war experiences. However, the PTSD label goes beyond combat experience to describe any person whose experiences leave him or her with profound feelings of fear, terror, and helplessness (American Psychiatric Association, 2000). Again, it is important to separate an event from the experience of it; some veterans experienced trench warfare, hand-to-hand combat, and sniper attacks without becoming severely traumatized. For them, these events did not become traumatic experiences. For others, the events led to traumatic experiences and continued to haunt these veterans long after the conflict ended. The first group may have experienced fear but not terror, while the second group experienced both fear and terror and, later, helplessness and shame.

Feelings of terror differ from feelings of fear. Most individuals experience fear from time to time; but usually overcome that feeling and get on with their lives. However, terror is much more intense and longer-lasting than fear. An individual's capacity for action may be blocked, making it difficult for them to effectively decide what to do or what decision to make. This state of helplessness is associated with the feeling that they are "terrorized" and feel frozen, becoming incapable of deciding, thinking, or appropriately reacting to a challenging situation, or even to an everyday event requiring a choice or decision.

Terror, shame, and helplessness are three of the hallmarks of PTSD. Betty, who we described earlier, was traumatized by her father's abuse for several years. Even after her father's death, she bore the physical and emotional scars of his repeated beatings. Eventually, the physical scars disappeared, but the emotional wounds remained.

The term "horror" is sometimes used to describe feelings associated with PTSD, but that term is less appropriate than "terror," even though both are associated with fearful stimuli. "Horror" usually describes a short-term abhorrence or loathing, not a long-term condition such as that accompanying PTSD. In addition, "horror stories" typically deal with supernatural fantasies, while accounts of "terror" describe people's reactions to real-life events. Finally, "horror" is derived from the Latin word *horrore*—to shake or shudder—while "terror" is derived from *terrere*, to frighten. Although we will use both terms throughout this book to describe the moods and experiences of people diagnosed with PTSD, we will not use them as synonyms.

"Shame" comes from a Scandinavian term implying disgrace and dishonor. In some cultures, the shame that accompanies PTSD is an extremely severe symptom because of its social connotations ranging from embarrassment to humiliation. Shame damages one's opinion of oneself especially as the PTSD survivor imagines how one's behavior displays failure, weakness, and a loss of dignity and social status (Budden, 2009).

Because such a variety of symptoms may occur, the advent of PTSD following traumatizing events varies from individual to individual. A traumatic experience can be defined as a life-threatening incident or injury that overwhelms the individual's capacity to cope with or integrate it (APA, 2000), an experience that challenges one's existential worldview (Beck & Emery, 1985). In the latter instance, the experience need not be life-threatening; taunting, teasing, and bullying, for example, may be traumatic even though they do not necessarily lead to physical danger (McNally, 2003, p. 233). These experiences may, however, drastically disrupt one's view of the world as a friendly place in which one is welcome and secure. They often result in shame, and a loss of status among one's peers—an outcome that can be devastating to adolescents.

These terms can be better understood by examining the historical and current implications of PTSD in survivors of such experiences as family violence (including spousal assault as well as child abuse), sexual abuse (perpetrated by either family members or strangers), involuntary sex trafficking (such as being forced into prostitution, escort services, pornography, and even cyber-sex), kidnapping, forced captivity, harassment, torture, life-threatening injury or illness, or armed conflict. But PTSD can also be associated with natural disasters; although the traumatizing event may not result in physical injury, it may involve the loss of one's home, witnessing the death of others, or seeing a frightening panorama of buildings being swept out to sea or being destroyed by a conflagration, fire, or inferno. PTSD also may follow automobile or motorcycle accidents, airplane crashes, entrapment in mining disasters, or human-caused stressors such as toxic spills or nuclear accidents. There is a real or perceived threat to life and physical well-being in each of these cases that may give rise to traumatization.

PTSD is not a new disorder; although the term was adopted as an official diagnosis by the American Psychiatric Association only in 1980. *DSM-III* described PTSD as a potentially sustained symptomatic response to a previous trauma, not as a reflection of "premorbid psychopathology." This linear, cause-and-effect view of PTSD as a result of trauma exposure alone was later criticized as overly simplistic, but it did represent a turning point in the field (Briere, 2004, p. 6).

Clearly, PTSD has existed for centuries, even though it has been described in different terms. The book of *Genesis* in the Bible tells the story of Isaac, who was bound, gagged, and nearly sacrificed by his father, Abraham, who thought he was following the dictate of Jehovah. Once Abraham's faith had been demonstrated to the satisfaction of Jehovah, Abraham was told to untie his son and sacrifice a nearby ram instead. Nonetheless, the Old Testament story goes on to relate how Isaac did not marry until the age of 40, when a bride was solicited for him. Isaac became embroiled in a dispute over the ownership of local wells and, in a cruel twist of fate, was deceived by his own son, Jacob, who stole his brother's birthright. In retrospect, one could make the case that the tale of Isaac, whether historic or legendary, concerns of a man whose life swung back and forth between passivity and social altercation, a key symptom of PTSD.

The historical account of Samuel Pepys's description of London's residents' sleep disturbances, anxiety, and angry outbursts following the conflagration of 1666 suggests unresolved reactions to trauma. Shakespeare's characters often underwent dramatic personality changes following trauma, ranging from Lady Macbeth's compulsive hand washing (following the multiple murders committed by her and her husband), to Hotspur's social isolation and sleep talking after a bloody battle in which he lost several of his kinsmen.

The psychological and physical impacts of overwhelmingly stressful events (such as war, assault, injury, loss, separation, and suffering) have been recognized throughout history as reflected in various religious texts (such as the battles and persecutions described in *The Holy Bible, the Bhagavad-Gita,* and *The Holy Quran*), and various forms of artistic expression such as Picasso's painting of *Guernica*; Tom Greening's war poems (Paulson & Krippner, 2007); the diaries and memoirs written by survivors of Nazi concentration camps (Arons, 2003); and such U.S. films as *I Know Why the Caged Bird Sings* (child abuse), *Misery* (forced captivity), *The Deer Hunter, In the Valley of Elah, Brothers, Stop-Loss,* and *The Hurt Locker* (all dealing with war trauma).

## CONTEXT

As mentioned earlier, PTSD commonly affects people who have been exposed to a life-threatening event that is outside the range of their usual experience (APA, 2000). PTSD affects those people by impairing their functioning, rendering them helpless and overwhelmed in their ability to cope with or integrate such an event. In order to understand the development of PTSD, some context indicating the uniqueness of the events that contribute to its formation is needed.

Although understanding an individual's (or a group's) experience of a traumatizing event is crucial to consider when formulating a diagnosis, the context is also important in comprehending the relationship of the trauma itself and how it is experienced. As mentioned above, there are many potentially traumatizing events that might render someone susceptible to being diagnosed with PTSD. However, since PTSD was developed primarily in connection with war and combat experiences, our initial focus will be on wartime stressors, which will facilitate the appreciation of the diversity of experiences. The U.S. Civil War (more properly, the War of the Rebellion), the Spanish-American War, the two World Wars, the Korean Police Action and Vietnam Conflicts, and, more recently, the Gulf War (Operation Desert Storm) and the Iraq and Afghanistan wars (Operation Iraqi Freedom and Operation Enduring Freedom) all left a wave of PTSD diagnoses in their wake.

The complexities of wartime stressors (such as seeing comrades die, the inability to distinguish friends from enemies, and the constant hyperarousal regarding issues of safety and trust) have existed in every major armed conflict. Indeed, the impact of combat upon veterans can be traced back to the first descriptions of humankind at war. An early diagnosis was "Swiss Disease," as reactions to war were observed among Swiss combatants (Marlowe, 2001).

Clashing political issues fueled the U.S. Civil War, and a similar theme can be found among most other wars as well, the major exceptions being those fought over territorial disputes. The politics of the Civil War involved the spread of slavery, and it divided the United States into two entities: The United States (the Union) and the Confederate States of America (the Confederacy). There were over 10,000 military battles during the course of the Civil War, most fought upon open ground. Battles consisted of infantry, militia, and artillery employing a combination of bayonets, swords, and range fire with rifles, muskets, and cannons. Civil War battles gave the combatants a dramatic exposure to the death of their military comrades, which led to what was referred to at the time as "exhaustion" or, more poetically, "solder's heart." This exposure led to an increased number of physician-diagnosed cardiac, gastrointestinal, and nervous symptom disorders that marked the lives of Civil War veterans. These conditions shaped the awareness of how both exposure to the death of others and physical wounds themselves contribute to the development of traumatic stress (Pizarro, Silver, & Prause, 2006).

During the First World War, the condition was dubbed "effort syndrome" or "shell shock." It is important to note that physicians arrived at such physical disease diagnoses by listening to veterans' self-reports and in observing physical symptoms, with little consideration given to the psychological stresses evoked by war-related experiences. As awareness of the psychological and physical impacts of war increased, so did the diagnoses. Earlier terms were replaced by "combat stress reaction," "combat neurosis," "adjustment reaction," and—most commonly—"battle fatigue" or "operational fatigue" following World War II and the Korean Police Action. Freudian psychoanalysts used the term "war neurosis," since no organic basis for the symptoms could be found. They recommended psychoanalytic treatment for the condition, a process that was long and costly. More often, a military physician would simply tell an ailing veteran, "Go home and get over it" (Greer, 2005).

It was not unusual for veterans of World War II to experience "flashbacks" on anniversaries of their combat on the blood-spattered beaches of Normandy or Saipan. Half a century later, some veterans were still having dreams of Japanese suicide planes heading toward their ships, of seeing the mangled limbs of their buddies falling off their bodies when help was offered, or—during their waking hours—seeing maggots crawling out of living people's bodies just as they did during jungle fighting in the South Pacific (Stone, 1994).

Psychotherapists treating veterans of the Vietnam Conflict discovered that traumatic stress impacted each veteran uniquely, depending on the context of threat exposure and the combatant's reactions to the threat (Tanielian & Jaycox, 2008). If combat incidents, for example, were higher in intensity (as in seeing comrades being blown up versus dodging nearby mortar rounds), the number of mental health casualties tended to be greater. In addition, combat incidents were likely to produce more mental health problems than the experiences of veterans who had been working behind the lines.

Combat in Vietnam was unique in that one's adversaries often could not be seen, because most battles took place in dense forests, which provided cover for snipers and their firearms. The presence of defoliate gases such as Agent Orange, employed to clear the foliage, often obscured enemy activity. In many instances, soldiers encountered villages where they believed residents were not to be trusted, but should be assumed to be hostile. Many women and children were killed simply because solders could not tell which ones were friends and which ones were enemies. The resulting guilt would come back to haunt many of these veterans in nightmares and daytime hallucinations.

Another unique fact is that veterans who returned from the Vietnam Conflict were commonly not valued for their service and were shamed on numerous occasions, often being called "baby killers." "Homecoming" for many Vietnam veterans involved being met with hostility and rejection, often interpreted as an indication that, for them, "America was no longer beautiful" (Eisenhart, 1977, p. 5). Furthermore, members of the armed forces were often sent back to the United States one by one, rather than with their comrades, resulting in a lack of social support. Because of the many negative encounters on their return, many combat veterans had considerable difficulty adjusting socially and vocationally (Hoge, Castro, Messer, McGurk et al., 2004). Well-meaning friends and relatives did not know how to react to what they saw as bizarre behavior. The pre-war self-concepts of the returning soldiers conflicted with the post-service images of themselves, often leading to work-related difficulties, alcoholism, substance abuse, and other symptoms of PTSD (Baum, 2004; Finnegan, 2008).

Even so, historical scholarship has confirmed that psychiatric casualties occurred less often in the Vietnam Conflict relative to other wars. The rate of breakdown was 12 cases per 1,000 soldiers, compared to 37 per 1,000 during the Korean Police Action, and at least 28 per 1,000 during World War II (Dean, 1997, p. 40). Varying diagnostic criteria make these statistics suspicious, of course, but they still challenge the stereotype of the drug-addicted, suicidal, pathologically isolated Vietnam veteran that persists in many accounts.

Since the end of the Vietnam Conflict, with the exception of the short-lived Gulf War, there was no significant degree of U.S. troop deployment to overseas territories until the Iraq War (Belasco, 2007; Tanielian & Jaycox, 2008). Unlike Vietnam, where the draft provided a steady stream of recruits, Occupation Iraqi Freedom was fought by an all-volunteer army. Troops were deployed for tours up to 15 months at a time and sometimes redeployed for longer periods. This pattern created a high degree of tension for veterans in combination with the daily stressors of roadside bombs, improvised explosive devices (IEDs), suicide bombers, the handling of human remains, the killing of civilians thought to be enemies, seeing fellow soldiers dead or injured, sexual abuse of female soldiers (usually perpetuated by "comrades"), and the inability to bring an end to the violent situations resulting from ethnic and religious rivalries among Iraqis themselves (Hoge, Castro, Messer, McGurk et al., 2004).

Due to the increased number of combat stressors, these veterans were at a higher risk for mental health disorders such as PTSD and related problems as depression, dissociation, and suicide-proneness. Ireland (2005) reported that U.S. suicides from 2003 to 2005 included only 62 among Iraq and Afghanistan veterans, not significantly different from suicide rates in the general population. However, the statistics since then indicate that the suicide rate has increased. Kaplan (2006) reported that suicides are occurring more often than following other wars, and that these veterans do not usually commit suicide until they return home from their tour of duty in Afghanistan or Iraq.

Assessing the contribution of military or combat experience (e.g., IEDs, sniper attacks, blast explosions) to the development of PTSD has been hindered by the overlap of PTSD symptoms with those characteristic of other diagnoses, including anxiety-related disorders, drug dependence, antisocial personality disorder, and endogenous depression. These confound the diagnosis and veterans' willingness or unwillingness to report symptoms (Hoge et al., 2004). While the mental health issues provoked by war are not new, it is important to note that the prevalence of such difficulties in veterans and the need for greater services to meet them is greatest at time of war (Marlowe, 2001; Milliken, Auchterlonie, & Hoge, 2007; Rosenheck & Fontana, 1999).

Particularly prevalent in the Iraq War, but not uncommon in previous U.S. wars, are occurrences of traumatic brain injury (TBI). Sadly, TBIs are now commonplace in Iraq War veterans (Tanielian & Jaycox, 2008), largely because "blast combat" (based on explosives or IEDs) is a frequent weaponry tactic used by insurgents (Hayward, 2008). Blast injuries increase not only the number of deaths and the loss of limbs, but also the complexity of traumatic stress and PTSD. TBI is a common injury resulting from IEDs and the type of body armor being used. Since TBI is so common, appropriate measures to detect brain injuries have been developed and are continually being revised (Hayward, 2008). It is ironic that, as body armor has improved, more soldiers are surviving blasts than previously; however, their survival comes at a cost, namely, the presence of TBI with its attendant behavioral and emotional problems, such as outbursts of anger, struggles with expressing thought or action, or inappropriate responses (Pitchford, 2009).

In the context of war trauma, it is apparent that the well-defined battle lines characteristic of previous wars have given way, in Vietnam, Iraq, and Afghanistan, to chaotic battle conditions. The resulting "fog of war" has led to confusion, frustration, and a loss of cognitive control among service personnel that, in turn, have brought about the killing of innocent civilians and the deaths of U.S. troops by "friendly fire."

When their tour of duty ends, veterans returning from recent wars have missed the welcoming context associated with troops coming home from the battlefields of World War II. Even though the hostile context that awaited many Vietnam veterans has not been repeated, festive parades and celebrations have been absent as well. Medals for heroic actions in Iraq and Afghanistan have been few and far between, and the behaviors of friends and relatives often have been inappropriate, through no fault of their own.

Many veterans have to cope not only with PTSD, but with TBI and other challenges as well. Even in terms of those veterans who choose to enter counseling and psychotherapy, the Veterans Administration has been overwhelmed by requests and further hampered by necessary screening procedures that reject help for malingerers—those veterans who "fake" PTSD symptoms in an attempt to collect benefits. It is said that some veterans exaggerate their symptoms in order to take advantage of the benefits, while others hide their symptoms in order to advance their military careers. Both of these strategies make it difficult to estimate correctly the extent of PTSD and other war-related conditions.

### Diagnosis

As discussed earlier, wartime has been the primary influence behind the identification of stress reactions finally leading to official recognition of the condition now termed PTSD. The recognition and diagnosis of "exhaustion," as it was called during the Civil War, were seen essentially as physical fatigue, a natural response to terrifying war experiences. Since little consideration was given to the psychological impacts of war, "exhausted" soldiers were returned into battle. However, it was clear that soldiers' experiences during the Civil War were producing additional physical symptoms (such as startle responses, heart arrhythmias, and hypervigilance) beyond exhaustion, ultimately giving rise to the new diagnosis of "soldier's heart."

It was in 1952 that the first edition of the *DSM* (*Diagnostic and Statistical Manual of Mental Disorders*) came forth with the diagnosis of "stress response syndrome," later termed "situational disorder" in the second edition, published in 1968. These terms were not limited to combat-related stress, but incorporated the effects of other traumatic experiences as well. PTSD was officially included in the diagnostic literature with the publishing of the *DSM-III* in 1980. The *Diagnostic and Statistical Manual of Mental Disorders, 4th Edition*, appearing in 1994, extended its definition of PTSD stressors, expanded its conceptualization of symptom-clusters, and amended its criteria to address symptomology in children.

The "final text revision" of the American Psychiatric Association's *Diagnostic and Statistical Manual*, which is abbreviated "*DSM-IV-TR*" (APA, 2000), documents the most updated criteria according to which a person qualifies for a diagnosis of PTSD. By understanding these criteria in context with the experience of the individual (not just in reference to the manual), practitioners can begin to understand their clients and the ways their attitudes and behaviors may be influenced by the disorder. Rather than just narrowly applying the *DSM-IV-TR* as a labeling system, a wise clinician will realize that PTSD is not to be seen in black-and-white terms, but in various shades of gray.

According to the *DSM*, the label of PTSD can be assigned only to individuals who have been exposed to events that have left them with such emotional residues as a sense of terror and feelings of helplessness. The person so diagnosed must manifest specific symptoms including intrusive imagery, hyperarousal, numbing, poor concentration, anxiety, and nightmares (APA, 2000). Further, a diagnosis of PTSD must be considered carefully, as its manifestation varies in individuals from different cultures who have been exposed to different types of traumas (Brown, 2008; Krippner & McIntyre, 2003).

Because the Vietnam Conflict was a major factor in PTSD being recognized as a disorder, a significant number of people have come to associate PTSD with war experiences. However, as should be clear by now, the disorder can result from any experience or set of experiences that impacts a person to the point where he or she is left with feelings of severe terror and helplessness. As previously discussed, it is important to note that feelings of terror differ significantly from other anxiety-related feelings. Human beings are genetically programmed to experience fear through the *fight or flight* response (Levin & Nielson, 2007). In contrast, when people experience terror, their fight or flight response shuts down, leaving them unable to choose what to do; instead, they feel incapable of deciding, thinking, or reacting appropriately. A common response is, "I freeze every time I need to make an important decision."

For example, the violence, terror, and carnage experienced on the battlefield may remind combatants that human existence inevitably ends with death (Solomon, Greenberg, & Pyszczynski, 2003). At the same time, watching an enemy combatant die can evoke a feeling of satisfaction, despite the possible emotional scarring that may later result from this experience. However, witnessing the death of a comrade exposes soldiers not only to the reality of their own vulnerability, but also to the wound caused by losing a bond to their unit (Fuchsman, 2008). This break has been especially evident in the Iraq war, since units are kept together throughout their tours of duty.

### Diagnostic Criteria

There are six criteria required for an individual to qualify for the diagnosis of PTSD: (1) An exposure to a traumatizing event that endangered one's physical integrity, threatening death or serious injury, evoking a response of helplessness and/or terror; (2) a persistent re-experiencing of the event (as defined by three or more of the *DSM* symptoms); (3) persistent avoidance and emotional numbing (as defined by two or more of the *DSM* symptoms); (4) recurring symptoms of increased arousal not present before exposure to the traumatizing event; (5) a duration of symptoms lasting for at least one month; and (6) the impairment of major areas of functioning (social, vocational, etc.) due to the experience (APA, 2000). All criteria must be met in order for a diagnosis of post-traumatic stress disorder to be considered. A detailed outline of the *DSM-IV-TR* criteria for the diagnosis of PTSD can be found at the end of this chapter.

### Exposure

Post-traumatic stress disorder can occur at any age, including childhood. An individual's encounter with a potentially traumatizing event is affected by its intensity, immediacy, and extent. There is some evidence that social supports, family history, childhood experiences, personality and physiological variables, and pre-existing mental disorders may predispose the onset of PTSD (Paulson & Krippner, 2007). However, PTSD can develop without any apparent predisposing conditions, especially if the experience is particularly severe.

The person experiencing the potentially traumatizing event is often referred to as the "experiencer." The initiation of PTSD relies upon the experiencer's exposure to a traumatizing event and his or her reaction to that exposure. This reaction must involve the direct experience of another person's death, or the actual or threatened death or serious injury (physical or psychological) to the experiencer or a person being witnessed by the experiencer. This can sometimes include learning about an unexpected or violent death, serious harm, or threat of death or injury of another person, even someone not emotionally close to the experiencer. (Sometimes, this is referred to as "secondary PTSD.")

For a diagnosis of PTSD to be applied, the experiencer's response must entail intense fear, helplessness, or terror (such as agitated or disorganized responses in children). Responses to the trauma typically include persistent re-experiencing of the traumatizing event, persistent avoidance of reminders associated with the trauma and numbing of responsiveness, and persistent symptoms of arousal. This latter condition is often referred to as "hyperarousal," as when an experiencer is startled by a loud noise in an environment that is free of IEDs or similar weapons.

Symptoms of PTSD can have a varied onset and duration, different for each person. In the case of individuals who have been experiencing symptoms for three months or less, they are said to be *acute*; longer than three months is considered *chronic*, but, if symptoms present themselves for the first time at least six months after the traumatizing event, they are considered to be *with delayed onset* (APA 2000). This sequence of symptoms corresponds with the triad described by Paulson and Krippner (2007) as the "predisposing, initiating, and maintaining" aspects of PTSD. Paulson and Krippner's PTSD spectrum is reflected in the contrast between chronic and acute PTSD.

As previously discussed, although the history of PTSD has been documented primarily in war veterans, the effect of traumatizing events varies, based strongly upon how a person experiences the event. Like the Greek philosopher Epictetus cited in Chapter 1, the Roman philosopher-emperor Marcus Aurelius observed that it is not what has happened to a person externally that is as crucial to the outcome as that person's internal reaction to what has happened. Therefore, we have found it useful to use the word "event" to describe the actual occurrence, such as the sudden death of a loved one, and the word "experience" to describe a person's reaction to that event, such as an extended period of mourning following that death, perhaps one marked by social isolation, insomnia, and inconsolable grief. Some traumatizing events affect entire groups of people. Mass displacement during periods of famine, floods, and warfare, as well as persecution, oppression, and genocide, often is traumatic to the survivors.

The 2001 terrorist attacks on New York and Washington, D.C., were severely traumatizing for many of the experiencers. There were 20,000 Pentagon employees who probably took it for granted that their building was impregnable. Before September 11th, the Pentagon did not have a single full-time psychologist on its staff; after the attack, it employed about 100 to provide help for workers who reported stress, anxiety, or depression. But instead of introducing themselves as therapists, they called themselves members of the "critical incident stress-debriefing team." Their handouts emphasized the fact that emotional reactions are not a sign of weakness, but a normal, expected reaction to a massive unexpected event. This immediate intervention probably prevented the onset of PTSD among any number of the Pentagon workers, one of whom commented, "For the first time in our lives, we feel vulnerable. It's as if our house has been robbed" (Goldstein, 2001, p. 84).

As mentioned previously, the diagnosis of PTSD was based upon a Western contextual frame of reference. Thus, it is extremely important to consider all possible elements of influence within a person's experience (ethnicity, age, gender, life encounters, and spiritual perspectives) before making a diagnosis of any kind. Oftentimes when people endure ethnic persecution, oppression, or displacement the proclivities for long-lasting, chronic PTSD are higher, especially if endured along with abuse, torture, or other threats to one's physical or psychological integrity.

### Re-experiencing the Trauma

Re-experiencing the traumatizing event is a key diagnostic cluster. It encompasses recurrent intrusive thoughts about the event, nightmares about the event, and spontaneous flashbacks in which the event is relived (McNally, 2003). The nature of the experience surrounding the event is the primary influence of how it might be re-experienced. For example, for some people, the re-experiencing might include flashbacks, nightmares, intrusive pre-sleep and daytime imagery, or intense recollections in which the event is re-engaged (Krippner & Paulson, 2006).

It is important to note that children have difficulty associating the experiencing of trauma to previous encounters. Rather, the re-experiencing takes the form of a constant, continuous, present threat. Thus, a common re-experiencing of abused children might include monsters attempting to harm them in dreams or disorganized and angry outbursts during the day, often accompanied by such physical symptoms as nausea, headaches, and lethargy.

Depending again on the nature of the person, he or she may find the overall re-experiencing so overwhelming that the distress evoked may cause significant cognitive impairment including dissociation—the disruption of one's flow of attention. The re-experiencing ranges in duration from individual to individual, but is felt to be real and relived upon its onset. Sometimes re-experiencing may occur without provocation, but in most circumstances, environmental cues (often called "triggers") similar to the original event signal the recollection, causing significant impairment to one's functioning. Some cues or triggers might be as subtle as recognizing a familiar smell, being in a crowded street, or even hearing a loud noise that resembles the traumatizing event or events.

Advances in neuroscience have made it possible to chart brain reactions during flashbacks. A team of psychiatrists at the University of Western Ontario studied 11 persons who developed PTSD as a result of sexual abuse, sexual assault, or a motor vehicle accident, and 13 persons who had experienced the same events without developing PTSD. All the participants in this study were instructed to recall the event while their brain activity was being monitored by a process referred to as fMRI functional Magnetic Resonance Imaging. In addition, functional connectivity analyses were made; together, these processes permit assessment of a network of neurons across several areas of the brain.

There were notable differences between the two groups of participants. Those with PTSD showed more activation in certain right-brain areas such as the right posterior cingulated gyrus, the right caudate, the right parietal lobe, and the right occipital lobe. Participants without PTSD showed more activation in certain left-brain areas such as the left superior frontal gyrus, the left caudate, the left parietal lobe, and the left insula. One does not have to know the location of these areas to observe the spectacular difference between the participants' brain activity (Lanius et al., 2004).

Flashbacks are usually visual in nature, extremely vivid, and fairly unpredictable. The right parietal lobe is known to be involved in non-verbal memory; thus its activation while people with PTSD are remembering distressing events may explain why these events are recalled as flashbacks. In contrast, the left-brain areas activated by the non-PTSD participants when they recollect disturbing events are consistent with verbal episodic memory retrieval and may explain why they remember these events as verbal narratives rather than as visual images. In addition, when these right-hemisphere areas are activated, people are less capable of taking in new information. As a result, they have difficulty making sense out of the traumatizing event and integrating it with other memories (Arehart-Treichel, 2004).

### Avoidance and Numbing

Individuals who endure traumatizing events often avoid venues similar to or reminiscent of the original settings. For example, if a young woman was raped in an alley in a downtown area of a city, she may avoid going to the city at all or simply stay away from dark areas. She may even refuse to go out at night. These trauma survivors try to avoid any type of reconnection to the trauma (including dialogue, thoughts, feelings, and memories). Other efforts to avoid and numb might include the abuse of illegal and/or legal substances, social isolation, or such psychological reactions as anger, amnesia, or so-called "conversion reactions," including blindness, deafness, or paralysis. These strategies help to numb the re-experiencing of any discomfort associated with the trauma.

Often automatic in response, emotional numbing can take place immediately following the traumatic experience and may include disconnection from usual and pleasurable encounters such as social activities, intimacy in relationships, vocational employment, or the expression of moods or feelings. Numbing of this nature is regarded as a diagnostic cluster of PTSD, along with re-experiencing the traumatizing event and various disturbances in thinking and planning (McNally, 2003, p. 231).

## Clinical State

Several studies demonstrate that people's current clinical state affects how they remember a traumatizing event (McNally, 2003, p. 233). A longitudinal study of Gulf War veterans indicated that they later remembered their traumatizing events differently from how they had reported them two years earlier. Seven out of ten veterans remembered an event during a follow-up interview that they had not mentioned originally, one month after the war ended. The severity of PTSD symptoms at the time of the follow-up was predicated on the number of traumatizing events originally mentioned. In other words, veterans with greater PTSD severity tended to amplify their memory for traumatizing events over time (Southwick et al., 1997).

In contrast to benign memory distortion, there have been cases of deliberate malingering and exaggeration of symptoms among veterans in order to obtain a PTSD diagnosis and the supposed financial benefits associated with it. Veterans who obtain a high service-connected disability rating are eligible for thousands of dollars per year, tax-free and adjusted for inflation. However, the financial loss is substantial, should they recover from PTSD. There are even cases where veterans who never saw combat or applicants who never even served in the armed forces have applied for PTSD benefits (McNally, 2003, p. 235). This problem is not confined to veterans; the risk of malingered PTSD arises in civil suits following accidents in civilian life as well (Rosen, 1995). On the one hand, mental health practitioners are eager to provide services for veterans who are reluctant to apply due to fear their service record will be tarnished. On the other hand, the practitioners need to be on guard against those who are all too eager to apply for services, looking for financial gain.

Not all PTSD stories end badly. Here is an account of a marine named Daryl Paulson, who enlisted in the U.S. Marine Corps in the late 1960s. He was consumed with patriotism and wanted to do his duty for the United States, feeling that he could make a positive difference by fighting communism while having an adventure at the same time. Paulson had grown up with an interest in firearms, had gone hunting, and had kept in shape by hiking through the mountains of Montana, his home state. His opportunity to use weapons came in 1968 and 1969, the years of the Vietnam Conflict's heaviest fighting. Assigned to the First Marine Division's Fifth Regiment, he participated in combat operations in the dreaded A Shau Valley, in the Antenna Valley, and in the so-called Arizona

Territory. Many of his buddies were killed in these operations and others were badly wounded.

Combat was not what Paulson had expected. It was exhilarating and exciting, but it was also physically taxing, emotionally draining, morally disturbing, and spiritually deadening. In Paulson's words,

> Ironically, the most damage to me occurred after my return from the war, when I reentered civilian life by attending college. There I was called a warmonger and a baby-killer. I became pretty much a reject from the larger community of my noncombatant peers. I found myself in complete and utter despair, unable to reintegrate into my culture. I had killed. I had killed with passion, and I had enjoyed the suffering that I brought to my enemies, for it was payback for what they did to us. Combat memories loomed over me during the day, and the faces of those I killed haunted me at night. My life became a cycle of suffering—and drinking to relieve the suffering. The cycle focused around drinking, and drinking, and more drinking. My life was not just a heap of images but a living hell many times worse than anything I had experienced in Vietnam. I was an alcoholic by my 24th birthday and dangerously on the verge of suicide. Unknown to me at the time, I was not alone in this dilemma. Years later, I discovered that every other person I knew in my unit also had descended into his own version of hell. It took me years of hard work to recover and to enter the social mainstream. (Paulson & Krippner, 2007, pp. xvi–xvii)

In mythological narratives, after the hero or heroine has successfully completed his or her initiatory experience, he or she returns to the world-at-large to share the newly acquired wisdom with members of the community in order to be of service to them. But for many of the returning Vietnam Conflict veterans, there was nothing of value they felt that they could share. There were only anguish, pain, and frustration. Instead of being treated as heroes, they were shunned by their former friends for their peculiar lifestyle; they were shunned by World War II and Korean Police Action veterans for having lost the war, by hippies of their own age for being warmongers, and by themselves for losing their patriotic ideals. Rather than being a war to save the United States, the Vietnam Conflict was a cruel turn of fate for those who fought it (Paulson & Krippner, 2007, pp. 100–101).

Paulson recalled,

> Plagued with guilt, I tried to find a place where I could go for forgiveness, to get away from this hell. I felt too guilty to go to God and church, for I had killed, I had injured, and I had tortured my fellow human beings with intense delight. No, I could not go to God or church, for I had too much blood on my hands. I reasoned that no one wanted me now, not even God, for I had killed His children. (Ibid., p. 101)

In therapy, Paulson began to work his way through the guilt that consumed him. By serendipity he read about John Newton, an English slave trader who, after experiencing a religious conversion, wrote the hymn "Amazing Grace."

*Amazing Grace, how sweet the sound*
*That saved a wretch like me!*
*I once was lost, but now am found,*
*Was blind but now I see.* (Newton, 1779)

Identifying with those sentiments, Paulson realized that he, too, could be forgiven. With that, he began to stop condemning himself and started to accept the fact that he had done the best he could do at the time. Further, Paulson resolved that he would not be a stooge again, putting his trust in people who supposedly know what is best. He began to take responsibility for his life (Paulson, 1994).

Paulson continues,

I began to accept myself for what I was, not as I should be. I recognized that while I was not the toughest person in the world, neither was I the weakest. I was not the smartest person, but I was not the dumbest, either. I began to accept my emotional sensitivity, ultimately even viewing it as a positive attribute. I gave up the idea that I had to be cold and insensitive to be a "man." I accepted that I had intention, creativity, and imagination, which I had considered character flaws at one time. . . . While it was difficult to do, I allowed myself, more and more, to be me—the authentic me. (Paulson & Krippner, 2007, p. 105)

Paulson went on to receive a PhD in psychology and to become president of the Bioscience Laboratories, Inc., a national testing laboratory facility located in Bozeman, Montana. He has used his firsthand experience with PTSD to counsel others, and serves as an example of what is possible when people enter therapy, take control of their direction, and start a new chapter of their lives.

### Betty Revisited

Briere (2004) has lamented that the notion of what constitutes a trauma is less straightforward than might be envisioned. In this book, we have attempted to resolve this problem by differentiating between an event, such as being in a motor vehicle accident, and an experience—the experiencer's reaction to the event. Some individuals recover quickly from a serious motor vehicle collision, even though it may have been life-threatening. Others may construct the sequel to the accident quite differently, having nightmares about it, refusing to enter a car again, or exhibiting a startle reaction when seeing two cars driving in close proximity on the highway, even if the experiencer is walking on the "safe" sidewalk.

The case of Betty exhibits another problem with the criteria offered by *DSM-IV-TR*, such as its inference that PTSD needs to be linked to a "single stressor" or to one traumatic event. Betty was repeatedly abused, and saw her mother's abuse numerous times. The threat of murder was an additional stressor, but *DSM-IV-TR* infers that the symptoms "must all occur in response to a single incident" (Briere, 2004, p. 8). Because Betty's symptoms cannot be linked to a "single stressor," some clinicians would diagnose her as suffering from an "anxiety disorder," even though her symptoms are strongly suggestive of PTSD. We, however, take the position that PTSD can be linked to either single stressors or to multiple stressors, either to single incidents or to multiple incidents. Betty's viewing of her mother's abuse was likely traumatic in its own right, as was her father's vow to kill them if they informed the outside world. Both incidents represented a threat to physical integrity, to health and well-being, and to life itself.

The case of Betty reminds us that clinical diagnoses are "social constructs," and as such they may vary from clinician to clinician and especially from country to country. But this recognition does not excuse the perpetrator of abusive acts or bring solace to victims of malicious actions. We need to note that the tenth revision of the *International Statistical Classification of Diseases and Related Health Problems*, published by the World Health Organization of the United Nations (1992), is more widely used worldwide than the *DSM*, even though its description of PTSD is similar. In addition, various indigenous folk healers might diagnose Betty as suffering from "soul loss," the theft of her essence by demonic forces who "possessed" her father, motivating his cruel and malevolent actions. We will, nevertheless, continue to use the *DSM-IV-TR* framework throughout this book, simply because it is the "only game in town" as far as mainstream psychotherapy in the United States is concerned. But we will also continue to draw attention to its shortcomings when it fails to do justice to specific cases. It is quite clear that each case of PTSD is unique, and it is a challenging task to find terminology that will do justice to individual differences. In the realm of PTSD, one size does not fit all.

# 3

# The Varieties of PTSD

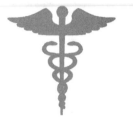

P ost-traumatic stress is a very complicated disorder. As noted in earlier
chapters, the American Psychiatric Association's *Diagnostic and Statistical Manual of Mental Disorders, 4th edition, Text Revision* (or DSM-IV-TR)
lists three main clusters of PTSD symptoms: (1) intrusive memories of the
trauma such as re-experiencing aspects of the event during both nightmares
and daily life; (2) emotional numbing such as the avoidance of social interactions, intimacy, and evasion of anything or anyone related to the trauma;
(3) hyperarousal and excessive nervous system activity including startle
responses, poor concentration, and psychosomatic disorders. The third cluster
of symptoms is marked by extreme anxiety and nervous tension. In fact, PTSD
is often considered to be an "anxiety disorder" (McNally, 2003, p. 229). It
follows that emotional numbing is a defense against the anxiety, while
re-experiencing marks the failure of a person's ability to cope with the anxiety.

Several films portray characters with PTSD who manifest these symptoms.
Hyperarousal can be seen in such war-related films as *Stop-Loss*, *Brothers*, and
*The Hurt Locker*. The latter film's protagonist displays a constant "charge" after
returning from his combat and disarming missions, and remains hyperaroused
and on "edge" when not in battle. At the end of the film, he leaves his wife
and child to return to Iraq, because combat affords him the best way of coping
with his underlying anxiety. Re-experiencing occurs in *The Town*, when the

leading female character has an intrusive image of her traumatic experience as a hostage following a bank robbery in which one of her friends was beaten senseless before her eyes. However, this seems to be a short-lived reaction and, as such, qualifies as an acute stress disorder but not as PTSD. Emotional numbing is the defensive maneuver used by Brick, the central male character in *Cat on a Hot Tin Roof*. The suicide of Brick's best friend was a traumatic experience for him, one that led to emotional numbing, primarily through alcohol.

Even so, traumatic experiences and their aftermath are quite difficult to describe accurately. Judith Herman (1997) astutely noted that the *DSM* does not do justice to what she terms "chronic traumatic stress," as when a child is confined for years by vengeful parents, or when spousal abuse permeates the entire duration of the marriage. Herman introduced the term "complex post-traumatic stress disorder" to describe these conditions, while others have used the term "chronic stress disorder" or "disorders of extreme stress" (Ozer & Weiss, 2004).

Herman also criticized what she saw as *DSM*'s failure to adequately consider an experience that threatens one's psychological integrity and worldview as traumatic. These traumatized individuals attempt to resolve the trauma internally, but their attempts are usually counterproductive. Herman observed in her book, *Trauma and Recovery* (1997), that in the aftermath of an experience of an overwhelming danger when "neither the intrusive nor the numbing symptoms allow for integration of the traumatizing event, the alternation between these two extreme states might be understood as an attempt to find a satisfactory balance between the two. But balance is precisely what the traumatized person lacks" (p. 47).

## THE COMPLEXITY OF PTSD AND RELATED PHENOMENA

PTSD is an ongoing reaction to one or more traumatic stressors. When we describe PTSD as an "ongoing reaction," we mean that, after a person's initial response to the traumatic encounter; he or she repeats the response or some variation of it. This is why the term "post-traumatic" is used; the traumatic stressor is not resolved, and one copes with similar life events ineptly or inadequately (Greening, 1997). For example, the ordinary stresses related to work, school, and/or relationships heighten the PTSD survivor's already existing stress responses. The results of this lack of resolution may include unemployment, dropping out of school, substance abuse, and divorce. Also, people's traumatic stress reactions can become exacerbated as the result of failed attempts at resolution, potentially leading them to "a sense of indifference and separation from the world they knew prior to [the traumatic event]" (Pitchford, 2009, p. 76).

Furthermore, this ongoing reaction complicates the symptoms, which become entangled with other life experiences. It is not enough for an accurate diagnosis of post-traumatic stress disorder to be made; there may be other conditions that contribute to the symptoms. People may have had previous stressful life experiences that can complicate how the diagnostician can accurately unravel the chain of events that led to the PTSD label.

There are many varieties of PTSD and Paulson and Krippner (2007) have placed them on a spectrum that ranges from mild to severe. At one end of the spectrum is "subliminal PTSD," in which stressors have not produced enough symptoms for a PTSD diagnosis. Individuals falling at this point of the spectrum have been exposed to stressors but have not been hospitalized, referred for psychotherapy or counseling, or sought help of any kind. A few symptoms are present, but not enough for a PTSD diagnosis to be made. However, later life experiences and the passage of time may evoke serious PTSD symptoms and a PTSD diagnosis. Also on the spectrum are those individuals who show severe stress reactions, even though their stressors may not be considered to be traumatizing. Members of this group often react strongly to separation from a significant other, divorce from a spouse, and other difficult life experiences that are generally not considered traumatic. Because the definition of PTSD rests on one or more traumatizing event as the activating factor, members of this group have not been placed in the PTSD category.

Once again, we need to emphasize that categories and diagnoses are what psychologists call "social constructs," terms that are constructed by people who have the power and authority to place other people in groups that often reflect a certain bias or worldview rather than the lived reality of people's lives.

Many writers focus on "peri-traumatic factors," the aspects of a traumatizing event that occur at the time of its occurrence. How many months was a person held captive? What types of torture were employed? For how many minutes did a rape occur? What bodily areas of a bullied prey were injured? How many friends of a solider were killed in a bomb blast? But it also is necessary to review the factors that can cause someone to be more vulnerable to traumatization than others. There may be biological factors that create a vulnerability to anxiety and excessive excitation. For example, studies of individuals with PTSD indicate oversensitivity in those parts of the brain and endocrine system that control reactions to extreme stress. These neural and endocrinal systems generate, maintain, and shut down stress-related hormones in the face of danger—a central aspect of traumatizing events (Ozer & Weiss, 2004).

The hippocampus is one part of the brain connected to emotional regulation; it has been found to be smaller than average in both individuals with combat and abuse-related forms of PTSD (Schmahl, Berne, Krause, Kleindienst, Valerius,

Vermetten, & Bohus, 2009). Although it is difficult to separate cause from effect, studies of twins who had small hippocampae indicate a predisposition to traumatization. One of the twins suffered combat trauma and one did not. When the hippocampae were examined, no differences were apparent following combat trauma. If trauma had "shrunk the brain," there would have been a difference between the twin siblings' hippocampae. Therefore, one could conclude that a small hippocampus may constitute a pre-existing vulnerability factor to PTSD (Gilbertson et al., 2002), or what Paulson and Krippner (2007) refer to as a predisposing factor for PTSD.

However, some physiological differences have been recorded. In a large-scale study, a comparison of veterans with no history of PTSD to those with a PTSD diagnosis found that the former manifested increased heart rate, facial muscle activity, and diastolic blood pressure (Keane et al., 1998). Skin conductance was also measured in these veterans, revealing an increased level of physical and psychological arousal as measured by the means of monitoring the electrical conductance produced by skin moisture. However, there were many exceptions to the general findings due, perhaps, both to individual differences and the possibility that some of the 778 veterans who were examined had successfully faked their symptoms to obtain a PTSD diagnosis for monetary purposes (McNally, 2003, p. 236). But the above-mentioned symptoms could be pre-existing, predisposing factors as well. A study of civilian trauma survivors found that elevated heart rate predicted subsequent PTSD (Shalev et al., 1998).

Extremely stressful childhood experiences also increase the likelihood for the development of PTSD later in life. Some children are ritually abused because their family has joined a religious cult; others are subjected to constant belittlement and criticism; still others have parents who espouse dogmatic religious beliefs and will abuse a child "to beat Satan out of him or her." Family histories of mood or anxiety disorders as well as unstable family situations during childhood have been linked to PTSD onset in later years (McNally, 2003, p. 238).

### Experience, Events, and Personal Myths

Once again, let's review the terms "experiences" and "events." An earthquake is an event, because an event is something that can be observed, measured, and reported by a number of people. But individuals will respond to this event in many different ways. Some people experience an earthquake as a dramatic life experience, one that they will talk about to other people for years, perhaps with a few embellishments. Other people live in a part of the world where tremors and small earthquakes are so frequent that they hardly bear mentioning in daily conversation. For still others, earthquakes are terrifying occurrences, and are often perceived as life-threatening. For months or even years, members of this group will have nightmares about the earthquake and may carefully avoid visiting earthquake-prone areas of the globe.

An event usually is a shared incident; it is something that people have in common. But each participant or onlooker may experience that event in a different way. What is stressful for one person may be run-of-the-mill for another. Therefore, we have used the term "traumatizing event" to describe what is extremely stressful for a particular person; we use the term "traumatic experience" to refer to a person's subjective reaction. For people who are so predisposed, a traumatizing event can become a traumatic experience. For others, it is a life event, often one they will long remember, but not a traumatizing event. It is a potentially traumatizing event because it can lead to a traumatic experience for some people but not for others.

Stressors are only traumatizing when they are perceived as such by an individual. Feinstein and Krippner (2008) used the term "personal mythology" to describe one's statements and stories about vital, existential life issues and concerns; personal myths are living narratives that have consequences for people's behavior. Like cultural myths (the *Bhagavad-Gita*, the *Odyssey*, the *Beowulf* saga, and *Quetzalcoatl's Journey*, to name a few), personal myths dictate morality, discriminate friends from enemies, define gender roles, and determine whether a life event has the power to traumatize the experiencer, often indefinitely. Homer's portrayal of the Trojan War and its aftermath included accounts of bizarre behavior by the war's survivors that are reminiscent of PTSD. Shakespeare's plays are filled with characters who, in their reactions to battles, murders, and betrayals, suffered symptoms that could indicate PTSD, an example being King Lear's senseless meandering following his betrayal by two of his beloved daughters.

Personal myths can determine whether an event will become a traumatic experience for the experiencer. The stressful experience of an individual—let's call him "Rico"—may (or may not) become traumatic depending upon his reaction to the event. In part, this reaction depends upon whether Rico participated in the event, whether he witnessed the event, whether his friends told him about the event, or whether Rico heard about the event from strangers or saw it on television. For some people, simply hearing about an event is enough to evoke a mild traumatic reaction.

Traumatizing encounters are an extremely personal experience. Whether or not the stressor becomes traumatic depends on how severely an individual's perceptions, beliefs, values, and personal myths are threatened. PTSD symptoms are influenced not only by people's responses to the event, but also by how their family and friends react to their experience. These variables are not easily captured by mere observation; it can be difficult to separate the specific elements connected to the traumatizing event from pre-existing features and predisposing conditions.

Traumatizing events used to be defined as unnatural or outside the range of usual human experiences (American Psychiatric Association, 1980). Herman (1997), however, suggested that traumatizing events are extraordinary not because they occur rarely, but "because they overwhelm the ordinary human adaptations to life" (p. 33). Being bullied, for instance, is a common experience in the United States; it is estimated that one out of six pupils is bullied at least once every school year. A high school clique of European Americans may torment and tease girls and boys whose African American parents cannot afford to buy them clothes that reflect current fads and fashions. A European American boy might internalize these taunts by saying to himself, "They are bullying me because I am poor." But an African American boy might tell himself, "They are bullying me because I am poor and black." An African American girl might think to herself, "They are teasing me because I am a poor black girl." And a gay African American girl might conclude, "They are taunting me because I am a poor black lesbian."

In truth, the bullies might be "equal-opportunity offenders," teasing anyone who is not dressed in ways that conform to the latest fashions. Some girls and boys will shrug off the remarks, knowing that the taunts are the product of immaturity and ignorance. But others will take the teasing behavior to heart, thinking about it constantly and internalizing it until it erupts in violent acting out, poor grades, prolonged school absence, or even suicide. In these cases, bullying becomes traumatizing, evoking a number of PTSD symptoms, some of which can have dire consequences.

### The Importance of Differential Diagnosis

Even though no two people experience trauma the same way, their symptoms may resemble the symptoms of other disorders. If not carefully considered and understood, an accurate diagnosis might be missed. Psychotherapists refer to this process as "differential diagnosis," because the specialist or specialists doing the diagnostic review (or workup) look for differences, distinguishing one disorder from others that might have similar signs and symptoms. For example, a person with PTSD may manifest depression but not be bipolar, might hallucinate but not be schizophrenic, might dissociate but not have a dissociative disorder, or might, at times, lash out at friends and associates, but a diagnosis of anti-social personality disorder would miss the mark. In addition, differential diagnosis, if done properly, will identify people who exaggerate or fabricate their symptoms in order to obtain financial compensation for their alleged "disability" (Burkett & Whitley, 1998).

Differential diagnosis is especially important for people who have endured multiple traumas over a long period of time, such as those whose background includes domestic violence. Their symptoms may resemble those of schizophrenics because they often exhibit paranoia, hallucinations, and delusions. Actually, they may have been trying to protect themselves from repeated trauma by becoming suspicious of other people's motives, by mistaking a compliment for an insult, or by confusing a toy for a weapon. If an individual is not accurately diagnosed for PTSD, this error could lead to an incorrect label and a therapeutic treatment based on that label that would do more harm than good, especially if medication is prescribed.

In addition, every symptom that occurs in individuals exposed to a traumatizing event may not be connected to PTSD. For example, some people, in comparison with others, are more anxious (manifesting hyperarousal), often avoid social activities (demonstrating avoidance), and disconnect themselves from their feelings (exemplifying numbing). These behaviors—by themselves—do not support a diagnosis of post-traumatic stress disorder. These symptoms might exist prior to a mugging, a sports accident, or being caught in a flood, and may even increase because of the event. But there need not be a cause-and-effect connection between a dreadful event and a subsequent increase in hyperarousal, avoidance, or numbing.

Quite often, there will be related diagnoses that need to be considered along with one's personal history. These may resonate with many points of the PTSD spectrum. Therefore, we cannot emphasize too strongly the importance of focusing on the experience of traumatized individuals in hopes of best capturing what they are living out within the context of their own unique world. The alternative is a "cookie-cutter" approach to their symptoms that ignores the potential variety of dissociative experiences.

### Disorder of Extreme Stress

As we discuss related stress disorders, we will use the terminology of *DSM-IV-TR*. This language uses words that, while often murky, represent the best terminology that mainstream psychotherapy has been able to evoke to describe these stress-related disorders and the devastating effects they have upon people. However, we are going to begin this survey with a term that does not appear in *DSM-IV-TR*, namely what several specialists refer to as Disorder of Extreme Stress (Ozer & Weiss, 2004).

People may not just experience one trauma, but multiple traumas. For example, someone might experience a traumatic response after enduring a motorcycle accident, but a short time later experience trauma again after the loss of a loved one. Again, the person's reactions to a stressor will determine whether the event is a traumatic experience for that individual. As mentioned earlier, a "Disorder of Extreme Stress" or a "Complex Post-traumatic Stress Disorder" frequently develops in individuals who are exposed to severe, prolonged, repeated trauma or several forms of interpersonal trauma. Examples would include prolonged torture, captivity following kidnapping, long-term domestic abuse, and imprisonment in a concentration camp (Herman, 1997).

The unique symptoms of Complex PTSD include ongoing struggles with one's identity, problems with maintaining one's psychological boundaries, sustaining intimate interpersonal relationships, and regulating one's emotional responses. Of course, they will manifest many or most of the symptoms of PTSD with an assumed single cause, such as intrusive imagery, nightmares, poor concentration, and avoidance of social activities.

Attention needs to be paid to this disorder even though it does not exist in the official *DSM-IV-TR* classification system. Individuals who are found experiencing symptoms of Complex PTSD are often diagnosed under the classifications of Disorder of Extreme Stress, Not Otherwise Specified. *DSM-IV-TR* uses the words "not otherwise specified" to suggest that traumatized people with severe identity and boundary issues deserve special consideration by psychotherapists because their symptoms are somewhat different from those characterizing people diagnosed with what is typically a single-trauma form of PTSD.

### Adjustment Disorder

What *DSM-IV-TR* calls an Adjustment Disorder is just what the name implies. These people have difficulty adjusting to life's challenges and stresses, but in contrast to PTSD, the stressor does not have to be traumatic. *DSM-IV-TR* cites six major adjustment disorders:

- Adjustment Disorder with anxiety
- Adjustment Disorder with depressed mood
- Adjustment Disorder with disturbed conduct
- Adjustment Disorder with both anxiety and depressed mood
- Adjustment Disorder with both disturbed conduct and poor emotional regulation
- Adjustment Disorder that is not easy to classify and is described as "unspecified."

PTSD is often misdiagnosed as Adjustment Disorder, because both are marked by anxiety that develops after exposure to a stressor. In the case of Adjustment Disorders, the stressor may not be severe enough to be regarded as traumatic. The distinction between the two disorders is that, with PTSD, the stressor is a traumatizing event, whereas with Adjustment Disorders, the stressor does not have to be severe. Furthermore, in Adjustment Disorders the stressor is usually a fairly common experience such as a series of family arguments, spending several nights in a dangerous part of a big city, or experiencing a long period of perilously rough weather on an airplane flight. Most people are able to rebound from these experiences in a short period of time, but individuals with Adjustment Disorders are not resilient enough to do so.

Donn had just finished college and was looking forward to taking a trip abroad with his friends. Prior to this trip, Donn had spent the last four years diving into his studies and spending a great deal of time working to finance this trip. He had never traveled far from home, having attended college locally and encountering little if any "excitement" during the 22 years of his life. But now, he declared, was the time for some excitement!

The day arrived and Donn and his friends decided to begin their trip by visiting a popular tourist location in Europe. However, this particular location was known to be a high-crime area, especially when tourists were in the vicinity. It was not long before a dozen young men stole all their purchases and threatened them at gunpoint if they called for police intervention. Donn and his friends ignored this threat and were shaking with fear when they filed a report with the local police. Once they returned to their hotel, they tried—without success—to get a peaceful night's sleep.

The next day, Donn's friends complained about losing the souvenirs they had bought; when they returned home, they described their "adventure" to their friends and families. But Donn was unable to assimilate the experience so easily. He continued to sleep fitfully, sometimes suspecting that someone else was in his house. He became suspicious of strangers and noticed that he was "on edge" much of the time. Fortunately, he saw a psychotherapist, who helped him to put the experience into perspective, and Donn's symptoms abated after a few months. When it came time to file for insurance reimbursement, Donn's psychotherapist diagnosed him as manifesting "Adjustment Disorder with Anxiety."

### Acute Stress Disorder

The difference between an Acute Stress Disorder and PTSD is that the former disorder shows up very quickly and tends to disappear quickly as well. The latter may not emerge for several months or even years, but then persists for a considerable period of time. To be labeled as someone with an Acute Stress Disorder, a person must have had active symptoms for at least two days and no longer than four weeks. If they last longer than four weeks, a PTSD diagnosis needs to be considered. The symptom clusters are somewhat different as well. Some degree of avoidance and arousal may be present with an Acute Stress Disorder, but there is more dissociation.

Marie had been working as a waitress at a local restaurant for over 10 years. She was a valued employee and was admired by the staff. Part of her duties included training new employees; so, when a new round of trainees was brought on, Marie assumed her responsibilities with great pride. However, she encountered some difficulties with one of the new employees who made sexual advances and groped her on a number of occasions. She finally reported his behavior, he was dismissed, and the sympathetic restaurant manager gave Marie a few days off with full pay. However, Marie became agitated and did not enjoy the period of rest and recuperation as much as she had hoped. When walking down the street, she often imagined that she was at an all-female spiritual retreat. When her imagined episode ended, she avoided walking near men who had any resemblance to the former colleague who had behaved inappropriately. She would even cross the street so she would not have to meet them face-to-face, even though they were complete strangers to her.

Marie's use of imagination allowed her to disconnect or dissociate from her experiences. Her dissociation continued when she returned to work. Again, she yearned for a spiritual retreat center or a private women's resort where the environment would protect her from any sort of major or minor sexual provocation. There was a women's discussion group in the neighborhood, and Marie started to attend its meetings. Quickly she discovered that the offense committed against her was minor in comparison to the rape, incest, and verbal and physical abuse reported by the other women in the group. She was embarrassed whenever she was called upon to describe her own experiences, because they involved no physical violence or coercion. However, the group leader told her to focus on her reactions and her feelings, as they were what needed resolution.

Marie discovered that she felt better when she spoke to the group. Her dissociative fantasies disappeared when she realized that she had found a setting that afforded her the safety of the fantasized retreat and resort. Once her symptoms disappeared, Marie continued to attend the group meetings, doing volunteer work such as answering telephone calls received by the group's "hot-line" service. The unpleasant incident at work and the Acute Stress Disorder it had inadvertently triggered added a positive new dimension to Marie's life.

In some ways, Marie and Donn had similar experiences. However, Marie's dissociation contrasted with Donn's anxiety. In addition, Marie's disorder was resolved in a few weeks, in contrast to Donn's disorder that lasted for several months. Some people with Acute Stress Disorder have symptoms that are more severe than those of Marie, so severe that psychotherapy is mandatory if there is to be a timely resolution. In these cases, if the symptoms persist for more than one month and meet criteria for PTSD, the diagnosis needs to be changed from Acute Stress Disorder to Post-traumatic Stress Disorder.

### Obsessive-Compulsive Disorders and Psychotic Disorders

Individuals with PTSD typically experience recurrent, intrusive images associated with the traumatizing event. This symptom resembles that of individuals impacted by Obsessive-Compulsive Disorders. The latter disorders are marked by intrusive thoughts, but these thoughts are not necessarily experienced in relationship to a traumatizing event. Some people are obsessed with cleanliness, compulsively wash their hands every hour, and have intrusive images of dirt, filth, and grime. They may even see stains on clothing that actually is spotless, or mentally enumerate the diseases they could contract from infectious food, kitchen utensils, handrails, or doorknobs. All of this could occur without the presence of a traumatizing event.

However, an Obsessive-Compulsive Disorder may co-exist with PTSD. Boris was in a church when a terrorist's bomb exploded, killing several members of the congregation. Boris survived, but developed the full range of PTSD symptoms. In addition, he manifested a compulsion to place chairs neatly in rows, mirroring the arrangement of the pews in the church before the bomb devastated them. Boris would invent various scenarios to explain why every chair had to be an equal distance from another chair. One time it was to accept a dare from a colleague; another time it was to make a mathematical estimate for a future meeting. The obsession was embarrassing, but could not be terminated until Boris entered psychotherapy.

Psychotic Disorders are far more serious as people with a PTSD diagnosis often report flashbacks and "relive" terrible episodes in their lives. These intrusions need to be differentiated from psychotic hallucinations, which are common among individuals impacted by the schizophrenias or so-called Brief Psychotic Disorders that do not require long-term hospitalization.

### Dissociative Disorders

When people dissociate, there is an interruption to the flow of their thoughts, their feelings, or their behaviors. They are no longer "in the here and now" because their attention has shifted elsewhere. Dissociation is a common peri-traumatic reaction (i.e., alteration of experience), as it defends the experiencer against the terror and anxiety of the immediate situation.

Angie was repeatedly molested by her brother. The first time he fondled her breasts and pubic area she was 14 years of age. Angie recalled later, "The feelings flew out of my body and did not return until several hours after the molestation stopped." Although peri-traumatic dissociation may serve an escapist purpose at the time of the trauma, it is a predictor of later PTSD (McNally, 2003, p. 239).

A person who repeatedly dissociates is said to have a Dissociative Disorder, one that interferes with everyday functioning. Spiegel (1984) observed, "It is not uncommon for individuals undergoing severe stress . . . to have at the time a spontaneous dissociative experience" (p. 110). The mildest of these is colloquially referred to as "spacing out," and the most serious as "multiple personality." The *DSM-IV-TR* refers to the latter condition as a Dissociative Identity Disorder because a person alternates between two or more identities and may not even be aware that such "switching" is taking place.

Dissociative Identity Disorder usually is associated with childhood trauma, but it may also arise in an adult. Duane was in his 50s when he sought treatment from Walter Young (1987), a psychiatrist. Duane reported finding that he had rented a hotel room in a distant city, would notice unexplained purchases on his credit cards, and would return from trips that he did not recall taking. A World War II naval veteran, Duane lost his wife because of his bizarre behavior. For example, he once left her for five months, at the end of which time he discovered that he was the district manager for 14 restaurants. Duane portrayed himself as "religious," and was appalled when unknown women would telephone him for sexual encounters or when he would awaken in a motel with a woman he did not know.

Duane described an inner voice that had talked to him since the war. At times, it merely told him to leave and get away from the "hassle," but at other times it encouraged him to commit suicide. When Dr. Young queried Duane about his pre-service years, he discovered that Duane's stepfather was an abusive alcoholic who repeatedly beat the boy's genitals and other areas of his body with a towel wrapped around his fist to avoid making visible bruises. During wintertime, Duane was made to sit naked in a dark coal shed for hours at a time to expel the "devil" from his "shameful" body. In fact, his stepfather would shave the hair off Duane's body in an attempt to purify him.

At the age of 16, Duane was sent to live with an older brother; there he joined a motorcycle gang and developed a close friendship with another member, Max. Duane and Max joined the Navy and served together at sea. While on duty, Max was killed in a tragic accident; Duane had told Max to take his stand at gunnery watch, while he left for a cup of coffee. Upon Duane's return, a Japanese airplane unexpectedly strafed the ship, mortally wounding Max, whose last words to Duane were, "I'll never leave you." Duane felt responsible for Max's death.

Dr. Young used hypnosis as a psychotherapeutic modality, gaining access to the identity named "Max." During one session, "Max" claimed to have "entered" Duane, holding him responsible for his death. "Max" admitted urging Duane to kill himself, as he had a score to settle, saying, "It wasn't my time to die." In the meantime, "Max" lived a hedonistic lifestyle, having sexual liaisons, riding motorcycles, and leaving home repeatedly.

Dr. Young observed increasing anxiety as psychotherapy proceeded, and Duane stopped coming for appointments after three months. His military records revealed that he had been misdiagnosed as "schizophrenic" while still in service; if Duane had been correctly diagnosed, proper treatment could have been initiated earlier and the outcome might have been more positive. Instead, he simply fell through the cracks and did not seek additional help.

The case of Duane underlines the importance of accurate diagnosis. Just as most cases of Dissociative Identity Disorder were misdiagnosed for many years, PTSD has been incorrectly used as well, delaying the beginning of appropriate treatment. Furthermore, PTSD often occurs in conjunction with other disorders, a situation that psychotherapists refer to as "co-morbidity." Dr. Young noted that Duane's condition contained elements of "pathological mourning," an attempt to maintain a lost object or person through identification with them. In any event, Duane's dissociative disorder prevented him from working through the painful guilt surrounding Max's death and he remains plagued by guilt and anxiety.

### Depressive Disorders

Depression is often a response to stress. If it was present prior to an exposure to trauma, it could become "with PTSD," in other words occurring along with PTSD. Briere (2004) accurately noted that "events severe enough to produce post-traumatic stress can also produce or exacerbate depressive symptoms" (p. 62). Oftentimes, the symptoms associated with depression appear as episodes of melancholy, sadness, regret, and ruminations on loss. Of course, these moods are part of the human condition, and there is a danger of pasting a "disorder" label on ordinary human experiences. Worse yet, moods of this nature can be "pathologized," and people who bring these complaints to their physician can be "medicated" and given a prescription for an anti-depressant drug. However, when the depression is severe enough to interfere with a person's ability to function in the workplace or in relationships, the term "disorder" is appropriate.

## CONSIDERATIONS AND RISK FACTORS

An individual's experience cannot easily be captured within the formal structure of a diagnostic system such as the *DSM-IV-TR*. The *DSM* often calls some of these factors "predisposing," meaning that they can increase the opportunity for stressors to evoke traumatic reactions. Paulson and Krippner's (2007) triad of predisposing, precipitating, and maintaining factors in PTSD illustrates the importance of these predispositions, whether genetic or environmental.

Such factors include (but are not limited to) age, ethnicity, gender, sexual orientation, previous psychological difficulties, family history, socio-economic status, coping patterns, genetics, and the subjective or personal distress caused by the traumatizing event. Any or all of these elements may increase or diminish the likelihood of developing PTSD when a person is exposed to stressors.

As noted above, the first criterion for a PTSD diagnosis is that a person has to have experienced, witnessed, or been confronted with an event or events that involve actual or imagined death or serious injury—or a threat to the physical integrity of oneself or of others. The response to that event (or events) needs to include intense fear, terror, shame, or helplessness. Again, this process is subjective and often difficult for an external observer, even a specialist, to identify.

Remember Marie? Let us examine her background more closely. Marie had endured difficulties in her attempts to secure work. She suspected that these difficulties were based not only on discrimination because of her gender, but upon the fact that she was unusually attractive. Whether rightly or wrongly, Marie felt that her job interviews were often marked by suggestive looks on the part of the men interviewing her, as well as flirtatious joking and sexist comments. As time went on, Marie became more highly sensitive to these innuendos and began to resent individuals whom she perceived to be the perpetrators of these offensive behaviors—in other words, the men in power.

These experiences predisposed Marie to experience Acute Stress Disorder when a fellow employee groped her from behind, not once but three times. She was correct in reporting the man who accosted her, and was pleased when he was dismissed and she was given a few days of vacation. But Marie was not resilient, and her background demonstrates how she was predisposed for the onset of Acute Stress Disorder.

Fortunately, Marie bounced back as a result of joining a women's support group, and her continued involvement with that group probably buffered her against having similar reactions in the future. Context is extremely important when attempting to understand traumatic reactions, and Marie's background provides data on predisposing factors that help explain her reaction to the activating incident. The resolution of Marie's disorder illustrates how the maintaining factors were handled in a productive way.

Some people can also develop PTSD reactions based upon what psychotherapists call "secondary" or "vicarious" exposure. Secondary trauma occurs when individuals are exposed to another's experiencing of a stressor. It involves an indirect exposure to trauma through a firsthand account or narrative of a traumatizing event. The vivid recounting of trauma by the survivor may result in a set of symptoms and reactions that parallel PTSD, namely, re-experiencing, avoidance, and hyperarousal (Zimering, Munroe, & Gulliver, 2003, p. 1).

For example, secondary trauma can occur among workers who respond to emergencies, such as firefighters, police officers, physicians, or other crisis response workers (Zimering, Munroe, & Gulliver, 2003). Since empathy is a natural human response, individuals may absorb the symptoms connected to other people's experiences of a traumatizing event, reliving them as if they were their own. As a result, it is important for crisis response workers to make provisions for adequate self-care through exercise, nutrition, healthy lifestyles, and social support.

Many potentially traumatizing events have been studied, revealing commonalities regarding what has allowed a trauma response to develop. Let's examine some of the common risk factors to better understand the complex ways in which stress and stressors interact with other factors.

### Age

There is more to age than meets the eye. Age is not only reflected in the physical development of a given person, but also guides how people relate to and understand the world around them. For example, a person's age can determine the social group with which he or she connects. These groups inform and develop the context and norms around life experiences that assist the development of personal myths about the past, present, and future. In relation to trauma, age can tell us how a person might experience a potentially traumatizing event. One's developmental stage reflects the possible intellectual and physical abilities available for coping with an unexpected event. Children and adolescents, for example, are more likely to experience stress reactions longer than do adults, until they become elders. Children, teens, and elders are more vulnerable to most types of trauma than adults, in part because they are dependent upon others for financial, emotional, and practical support (Brown, 2008).

A child who is sexually molested by a family member might be puzzled, but not necessarily traumatized. Once the molestation is discovered, the child becomes the center of attention and receives well-meaning emotional support. But this support can backfire, as the child suspects that he or she was the cause of the molestation, or that something "really bad" happened as a result of actions by an adult, often someone the child admired. Most teenagers, on the other hand, are more sophisticated about sexual abuse and its implications. If a trusted adult, such as a family member, teacher, or member of the clergy, perpetrates the abuse, the teenager's sense of trust is often violated, and his or her personal mythology about caring adults may be dealt a mortal blow.

Gary's minister repeatedly molested him as a child, and the molestation continued until Gary reached adolescence. At that time, he realized the implications of what had happened, and the event became a traumatic experience. During the ensuing trial, in the course of which a dozen other young men were called upon as witnesses, Gary recalled, "Once I realized that I had been used as a sex object, my whole world fell apart. I lost my religion, I lost my trust in adults, I lost my sexual identity, and I lost my direction in life." Gary's psychotherapist helped him deal with this existential crisis, but his peers who refused psychotherapy were not so lucky; within a few years, two had lost their jobs, one had been divorced, and one had terminated his life.

### Gender

You might think that gender is defined by the biological make-up or sex of an individual. However, sex is not just "normed" by genitalia. A person's sexual identity is also informed by social definitions and personal experiences. For example, what might be a natural expression for a young person can be considered by adults as "inappropriate" or "wrong." Sometimes young boys are bullied for being "girly." Their more "feminine" cohorts may challenge girls who are "tomboys." Such roles are imposed at an early age and affect the core development of one's identity. These young people might or might not take on the labels of "gay," "lesbian," or "bisexual" once they become sexually active. If so, they face more prejudice, discrimination, and—all too often—emotional and physical abuse. Sexual preference is not necessarily associated with unconventional appearance, behavior, and interests; hence many homosexuals and bisexuals are able to escape censure, at least until their "deviant" behavior is discovered or they are "outed."

Even more severe censure is directed against individuals who have been born "intersex," with genitals of both sexes, or who become "transgender," identifying with the opposite gender. The latter are more prevalent than the former, and are given special recognition by some societies, for example, people who Westerners refer to as "homosexual" or "transgender" were seen as one of the Great Spirit's rare creations among many Native American societies before Europeans arrived and branded their activities as "sinful" (Williams, 1992). However, in the United States both groups face discrimination and rejection.

Even though San Francisco is often seen as a "gay Mecca" for young people with diverse sexual orientations, surveys of the city's public schools indicate that gay slurs are rampant. With nearly four out of six of San Francisco residents being born outside the United States, many young people have parents from countries and ethnic groups that spurn gays, lesbians, bisexuals, and transgendered people just as vehemently as those from other parts of the country. One former student remarked, "Even though people assume this is a utopia for queer youth, it's very difficult . . . for adolescents who are beginning their life" (Smiley, 2010, p. 14). Even though there are "Gay-Straight" Alliance Clubs in high schools, some 82 percent of high schoolers in the city said that they have heard antigay remarks; only half the students reported hearing staff members or faculty stop students from making the remarks (Smiley, 2010, p. 15).

In 2010, Seth Walsh, a 13-year-old from Techachapi, California, hanged himself from a tree in his backyard following antigay bullying at his school. Rutgers University freshman Tyler Clementi jumped off a bridge after his roommate posted a video online of him in an intimate encounter with another male. Following these and many other suicides by traumatized young people who were taunted and ridiculed by their peers, Dan Savage, a well-known sex and love advice columnist, started a campaign focusing on the message "It Gets Better" (Savage & Miller, 2011). This gesture of support was endorsed by Laura Bush, Hillary Clinton, and other prominent men and women who want to reduce the risk factors for young people whose sexual history, gender identity, or personal lifestyles put them at risk for trauma.

An earlier attempt to protect these at-risk young people from abuse is The Laramie Project Initiative. In 1998, a young man named Matthew Shepard was brutally murdered because he was gay; the Initiative is named in his honor and has made videos, printed materials, and dramatizations available to high schools around the country. In 2011, the pop singer Lady Gaga's song "Born This Way" became an anthem for many bullied teenagers, one of whom wrote to her, recalling, "At every concert you've said that you want to liberate us, and that is what you've done. Your songs have taught me not to listen to haters and be who I am, because, baby, I was born this way!" (Savage & Miller, 2011).

On a broader scale, the risk factor for traumatizing events and stress responses varies with gender. Nearly half of U.S. adults experience at least one potentially traumatizing event in their lifetime (Schuster et al., 2001). However, 10 to 20 percent of women and 5 to 8 percent of men in the United States experience PTSD at some point (Kessler et al., 1995). Women are more likely to encounter relational violence than men, while men are more likely to experience combat-related trauma, although these proportions are changing as more men report spousal abuse and more women are exposed to combat (Kulka et al., 1990). Once they enter psychotherapy, women may have an advantage over men in integrating traumatic memories into their personal mythology and life narratives, and in verbalizing their memories. This may be related to male/female differences in the way the brain's hippocampus processes intrusive memories, where females seem to have an advantage (Saigh & Bremner, 1999).

Herman's (1997) feminist analysis of PTSD emphasized how social factors as well as individual reactions to upsetting episodes can induce trauma. She advocated civic activism as a counter-measure to the denial and repression that abused women often face. An example would be to match the legal definition of "sexual assault" to women's actual experiences, so that the violator cannot claim the incident was one of "mutual consent."

Herman made an astute observation: the increased attention given to PTSD in the 1970s paralleled the women's liberation movement as well as advocacy for children's rights. The perpetrators of trauma often use secrecy and silence to mask their activities, or attack a woman's credibility when she complains. Herman called for women to break this silence and underscored the importance of social support to validate their experiences, noting that persons in the survivors' world have the power to influence the eventual outcome. Some commentators have contended that, more than any other psychological disorder, PTSD forces consideration of political advocacy as a critical prevention tool (Ozer & Weiss, 2004).

### Social Class

Socio-economic status is a very complex area in the West and across the globe. Except for those cultures with well-defined caste systems, the intricacies involved are mostly invisible, embedded, and informed by social and individual perception and identity. Social class is defined primarily by financial income, educational level, and family background. Whatever group one identifies with is the lens through which others in the world are viewed. These perceptions can often lead to misinformed communications across the classes. For example, individuals living at the poverty level may see those whom they consider "rich" as happy, entitled, and disconnected from the harsh realities of life. Wealthy individuals might view those who are "poor" as lazy and not motivated to improve their circumstances. There are many inaccuracies in both views, but they inform the responses in both groups, which can often lead to bitterness and resentment.

In addition, life experiences can affect how a person enters a social class. Disability, for example, is often associated with fixed-income individuals. Even if the person has an advanced educational degree or comes from a "privileged" family, he or she may still be limited by a disability. Veterans with PTSD sometimes end up homeless, as do women who have left a marriage marked by physical and emotional abuse. Using data from the Panel Study of Income Dynamics, an annual survey of families and individuals conducted since 1968, MacLean (2010) discovered that soldiers exposed to combat were more likely than non-combat veterans to be disabled and unemployed in their mid-20s and to remain so throughout their work life span.

Social class may also affect one's ability to pay for adequate medical and psychotherapeutic care. Traumatic stress often requires high-cost treatments. If someone has limited financial resources, the access to care is diminished and can often raise the stress level. An additional financial burden is imposed if someone encounters legal difficulties related to PTSD. Examples would be physical assault, drug dealing, tax evasion, and traffic violations. One out of four Vietnam veterans ran into serious legal problems after their return, whether or not they had a PTSD diagnosis (Marciniak, 1986).

Social class can affect measured intelligence, both because of test questions that were standardized on more privileged groups and because low-income families have less access to books, cultural experiences, healthy nutrition, and other factors that affect intelligence. Lower intelligence test scores were associated with PTSD onset among Vietnam veterans; in tests taken before deployment, those who developed PTSD had average test scores, with an average IQ of 110. Those who did not develop PTSD had significantly higher scores, with an average IQ of 119 (Macklin et al., 1998).

Higher intelligence test scores were the best predictor of resilience against PTSD among inner-city children and adolescents who were exposed to such potentially traumatizing events as witnessing robberies, being caught in fires, and experiencing physical and sexual abuse. Among those with above average intelligence, 67 percent showed no signs of PTSD, but among those with below average test scores only 20 percent were free of PTSD or PTSD symptoms (Silva et al., 2000).

### Ethnicity

Ethnicity is often confused (or equated) with "race." However, ethnicity is not as easily observable as skin color or eye structure. Rather, ethnicity refers to a composite of tradition, culture, language, and heredity. Traditions are the customs and practices carried on over the generations within a particular group or society. Culture refers to the customs, traditions, values, attitudes, and social characteristics of a particular group. Language is the system of signs and symbols that is used for communication within that particular group. As a result, the label of "Caucasian," for example, does not exclude one from being a member of a variety of ethnic groups. And even when people have a family history from a country different from their residence, they may not identify with their original ethnic group. One example might be a family that emigrated from Russia to the United States during the early 1900s. The customs of their "homeland" were carried over to the new environment, but at the same time they were "acculturated" as Americans and their descendents called themselves "Americans" not "Russians," or even "Russian Americans."

The dynamics of family, personal, and cultural history, along with the intergenerational transmission of customs and behaviors, lays open the possibility for traumatic encounters to emerge, evolve, and be transmitted. Examples can be seen in cross-cultural marriages (e.g., Caucasian Asian) where there is an exposure to potential racial biases among families and cultures. Another example can be seen in individuals who assimilated into a culture only to learn much later in life about a family history of trauma. As a result, they might not be able to easily process the traumatic experiences that were hidden or ignored. For example, children of genocide survivors often know little about that experience because their parents have taken on a new culture and life. When the children do learn about their parents' traumatic history, they will sometimes develop PTSD symptoms themselves, as a sympathetic reaction to their parental history.

### Maladaptive Coping Styles

A coping style is one of many strategies people use to overcome difficult circumstances. Some examples relevant to PTSD might be self-care through nutrition and exercise, joining social support groups, engaging in sports and creative outlets, and participating in spiritual and religious practices. Maladaptive coping styles refer to impractical or harmful activities in which a person might engage, such as overeating, reckless driving, "cutting" and other forms of self-mutilation, engaging in promiscuous and unprotected sex, or habitual substance and alcohol abuse (including prescription medications). Life-threatening activities can be a coping mechanism for some, so it is important to understand the intention of the activity, especially when someone engages in such risky behavior as "extreme sports." Does the activity help or hinder the person's coping style? For many people with PTSD, the anxiety aroused by the traumatic stress is more than can be tolerated, so behaviors are evoked to help regulate that anxiety. For example, various legal and illegal substances might seem to help ease the anxiety associated with the stressor, but using them can often exacerbate the anxiety, especially when one begins detoxification. The anxiety that results may drive the individual to continue the behavior secretly.

It is not always easy to determine whether a specific behavior is maladaptive or adaptive, but clues can be obtained by examining a person's lifestyle. Signs of maladaptive coping are missing appointments or work, engaging in shallow social relationships, and demonstrating poor sanitary health habits. Because PTSD often occurs in conjunction with other challenges such as traumatic brain injury (TBI), this condition can impact a person's ability to develop adequate coping tools.

The most contentious issue in diagnosing PTSD concerns the accuracy of recovered memories of childhood sexual abuse. Some of the most respected figures in the PTSD field, Judith Herman among them (Herman & Schatzow, 1987), have suggested that children engage in "massive repression" that wipes out memories of the trauma until it is "recovered" in psychotherapy, usually by hypnosis. One team of writers has asserted, "Because some victims of sexual abuse will repress their memories by dissociating them from consciousness, hypnosis can be very valuable in retrieving these memories. Indeed, for some victims, hypnosis may provide the only avenue to the repressed memories" (Brown, Scheflin, & Hammond, 1998, p. 647).

However, children are typically confused rather than traumatized by sexual abuse (if it does not involve overt violence), so there is no need for "massive repression" to take place. They may forget the event simply because it was difficult for them to comprehend. Susan Clancy (2010) pointed out that it is not the abuse itself that causes trauma, but the narratives that are later imposed on the abuse experience. These narratives stem from negative social reaction to the abuse, so that the abused children may become adults who are intensely ashamed of their role in the encounters. Shame, in fact, is often central to the development and course of PTSD (Budden, 2009). In addition, McNally (2003) contends that experimental data in hypnosis indicate that not only does this technique fail to enhance the accuracy of recollection, but it can foster the production of "false memories" that are mistakenly experienced as accurate (p. 241). In contrast to childhood experiences, in the case of adolescents and adults, traumatic experiences are remembered all too well.

We introduced the term "co-morbidity" earlier; something "morbid" is "dark" and "gloomy," terms that describe many DSM disorders. When PTSD and TBI occur together, this co-morbidity presents psychotherapists, physicians, and occupational therapists with a challenge as well as an opportunity. But there are other problems that can exist along with PTSD, and psychotherapists need to engage in differential diagnosis to discover whether or not they are present (Mendelson, 1987). The challenge is one of accurate analysis; the opportunity is to encourage members of the helping professions to work together to rehabilitate a human being whose body and psyche have been shattered. Some Buddhist traditions view the path of healing through overcoming suffering as a form of spiritual practice at its highest level (Davies, 2011). If this is so, then working with PTSD is a way to mend wounded individuals, giving them an opportunity to live a better life and make their own contributions to society.

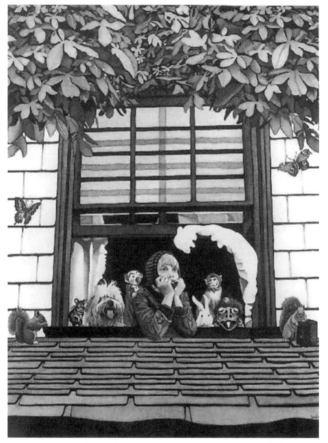

Stephen (Reproduced from the original art of Dierdre Luzwick.)

# 4

# PTSD in Children and Adolescents

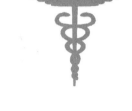

Hernando is a Mexican teenager with a history of PTSD. Since he has very eloquently described the traumatizing events that led to his condition, we will use his own words.

I was abandoned by my parents, but my grandmother willingly raised me. My cousin Alma and I had the pleasure of growing up with my grandmother; she loved my cousin and me so much. We were her favorite boy and girl in the whole world.

Grandma was always healthy; she had outlived three husbands and had seventeen children. I thought she would live long enough to meet my grandkids just like her own mom did. Her mom died at the age of one hundred and one, and I thought my grandma was going to live even longer. And of course I thought my great grandma would die before my grandma. My grandma refused to go to the doctors in Mexico or across the border in the United States because several times they had given her the wrong diagnosis about breast cancer. She never had it, even though they gave her that diagnosis twice.

One day she felt very sick. She lost consciousness, and one of my uncle's friends convinced him to bring her to a hospital in the United States. She got better for a day or two, but because of the doctor's negligence and the nurses' lack of attention my grandma's lungs filled with water and she fell into a coma. One of my uncles gave her mouth-to-mouth resuscitation, not letting her die right away, but after this we were told there was almost no chance of her surviving. When I heard this, I cried so much that I couldn't even go to school thinking that she was going to be gone when I came home. By the time she died, I had cried so much that I was like a zombie during the funeral service.

When the grieving was done, I couldn't stop blaming myself for not being with her for the last couple of months. I had been giving all my attention to school and to my pregnant girlfriend at that time. I began to have nightmares about my grandma in the hospital, begging for help and not getting it. My concentration in school was poor because I was thinking about her so often. Finally, I was just numb emotionally. I couldn't feel anything, even when I was with my girlfriend who was about to have our baby.

I was numb for an entire school semester and my grades suffered. I could not express feelings around my newborn son, and my girlfriend thought I had rejected him. We broke up and she found another boyfriend, one who was more responsive to her emotional needs. I was fired from my part-time job because I could not follow directions adequately. I saw my grandma in our house, in crowds, and in my dreams. Actually, my dreams were more like nightmares because they took place in scary hospital rooms, and my grandma was always in bed, wasting away, and sometimes turning into a skeleton.

I thought I was never going to get better. But I went to the school counselor, and she helped me get back in touch with my feelings. Unlike the other depressing and stressful situations I have heard of, this one made me a much better person. It helped me appreciate my family. It taught me not to be so cold, to show some emotion to my family, and every once in a while tell them how much I really love them. Once I was able to express my feelings again, the nightmares stopped, and I was able to do better in school. I feel like my grandma is taking care of me and always guiding me from up there.

Hernando's story represents a reaction to loss that developed into PTSD. Not every teenager who loses a loved one is affected this severely, but Hernando had experienced very little love in his life. This lack of affection predisposed him to PTSD once his beloved grandmother died. In this chapter, we present an overview of PTSD in children and adolescents, describe two additional cases, and provide in-depth material from researchers who have studied and treated PTSD among members of this age group.

## WHO IS AT RISK?

In addition to the loss of a loved one, potentially traumatizing events in the lives of teens might include physical, sexual, psychological, or emotional abuse or other violent incidents. Such events may be natural or human-made. The former would include floods, hurricanes, or earthquakes while examples of the latter would be bullying, ridicule, motorcycle accidents, or living in a war zone. Half of both Israeli and Palestinian children have nightmares at least once a week. Clearly, PTSD does not play politics! For example, the massacre of nearly two million Cambodians by Pol Pot and his group of radical communists traumatized the entire country. PTSD was investigated in a sample of 59 Cambodian adolescent and young adult refugees who had survived massive childhood trauma. Over half the group suffered PTSD at some point in their lives, and major depression and social phobia were found to accompany PTSD. Survivors who still manifested PTSD had the highest number of conditions, and those with no PTSD had the lowest (Deykin, 2002).

There are a number of child protection agencies in the United States ranging from those sponsored by the government such as the U.S. Administration for Children and Families, as well as private agencies such as the Massachusetts-based Child Trauma Institute and the New Jersey-based Summit Medical Group. Canada's Northwest Territories Health and Social Services performs similar functions. Agencies in the United States receive over two-and-one-half million reports per year involving over five million children and teens who needed some type of treatment. Many of these requests come in on the National Domestic Violence Hotline. Upon investigation, approximately 30 percent of these reports yielded results indicating harm, including neglect as well as physical, sexual, or emotional abuse (Osofsky & Lieberman, 2011). Also, millions of children witness family violence, with a high percentage involving child or teen physical abuse. Many cases go unreported. One boy was told by his mother, "If you dare tell the police that I am beating your father, I will kill you on the spot" (Chamberlin, 2010, p. 55).

However, it seems clear that rates of PTSD are higher for certain types of trauma survivors. For example, nearly all children manifest some type of PTSD if they see a parent being killed or if they witness a sexual assault on a loved one. Furthermore, PTSD develops in about 90 percent of sexually abused children, 77 percent of children who see a school shooting, and 35 percent who encounter violence in their neighborhood, even if they are not the target of the shooting or assault (Hamblen and Barnet, 2009). The rash of school shootings in the United States has had a negative effect upon many of the survivors. Children who had been most exposed to the threat of attack had the greatest number of PTSD symptoms. However, not all who experience such events develop PTSD. For one reason or another, some children are more resilient than others, while others simply lack the capacity for empathy, for putting themselves into the "psychological shoes" of a person who they see being abused or attacked.

Three main factors that can increase the likelihood for children and teens to develop PTSD include: (1) the severity of the trauma, (2) the parental response to the trauma, and (3) the youngsters' proximity to the trauma or to the survivors of the trauma. Those children and teenagers who directly experience a trauma tend to have the highest number of PTSD symptoms. If they are farther away from the event geographically, they report less distress. The symptoms may not be as severe if the child has a supportive family and if the parents do not over-react to the trauma by discussing it frequently, thus re-traumatizing the child.

Other factors can affect how PTSD manifests in an individual. Events that involve people hurting other people are more likely to result in PTSD than other types of trauma. Also, the more traumas a child undergoes, the higher the risk of getting PTSD. Some research indicates that ethnic minorities have higher levels of PTSD. This makes sense because of racism, discrimination, and stereotyping; children can be teased and taunted because of their skin color, their clothing, or their religious affiliation. As we have mentioned in the previous chapter, gay and lesbian teenagers can be mercilessly ridiculed, often to the point where they contemplate suicide, or actually end their lives.

Another question is whether a child's age at the time of the trauma has an effect on PTSD. Some researchers suspect that the effects of trauma do not differ according to the child's age, but that it may be that PTSD looks different in children of different ages. For example, an adolescent with PTSD may lock herself in her room for days, only emerging to eat and to use the bathroom. Few adults with PTSD would be able to behave in this manner, but might shun conversations at work, eat by themselves at lunch hour, and avoid social engagements on weekends (Carrion, Weems, Ray, & Reiss, 2002).

## THE IMPACT OF PTSD

There seem to be two types of trauma leading to PTSD symptoms among young people. One is characterized by exposure to a sudden, one-time event, whereas the other results from exposure to repeated events. It is likely that with each additional trauma, a child or teen's resilience becomes overwhelmed, leading to PTSD. No matter which of these two types is involved in PTSD, the condition in childhood and adolescence can affect normal development, often disrupting the acquisition of the skills necessary for a child to become self-sufficient. For example, throughout childhood and especially in adolescence, brain development occurs fairly rapidly. If a trauma were to be experienced, parts of the brain may slow or stop in their developmental process. When there is an occasion that demands a mature reaction, the traumatized teenager might resort to already established neural structures. In other words, he or she would step back into behaviors that would characterize someone younger than the child's actual age. This reaction, whether it be screaming, smashing, or running away, is simply an attempt to cope and survive the experience. It is the best response the teen can make, given his or her level of brain development.

For some psychotherapists, the "one time event" that can be traumatizing is birth itself. The pioneering psychoanalyst Otto Rank (1929) wrote of the "birth trauma," a concept that met with ridicule by mainstream practitioners who pointed out the that newborn child's nervous system was not mature enough to recall this event. However, Stanislav Grof (1985), a psychiatrist, revived interest in this topic by criticizing the "exclusive focus on psychological traumas," and presented a variety of scenarios in which different birth conditions could be traumatizing events (p. 96). Somewhat later, according to another school of thought, "separation trauma" occurs if a newborn baby is given up for adoption and is "relinquished" by his or her birth mother to live in a world devoid of genetic markings and "mirroring" (Verrier, 1993). These proposals are highly speculative but provide fertile areas for investigation; their proponents have provided a number of case studies that provide supportive evidence, at least in their appraisal.

In most instances, young people's responses to stress are brief, and they recover without exhibiting further problems. A child or teen exposed to a stressful event may assimilate that fight, taunt, or accident into his or her compilation of disagreeable experiences and not suffer undue aftereffects. However, as is true of what happens to adults, for the stressful event to be traumatizing to children or adolescents depends on how they relate to and perceive that event. The major difference is that a child's risk of developing PTSD is related to the evaluation the child brings to that event. Most adults have a broader perception of what constitutes life-threatening danger. Thus, a child might witness a domestic argument and think that one parent is about to kill the other parent. Sometimes children have seen similar events enacted on television, in the movies, or even portrayed in popular music. Translating this pattern to a real-life setting may not be logical to an adult, but may make sense to a child.

In addition, there seems to be general agreement among the medical and psychological communities that PTSD symptoms are quite different for children than they are for adults. Once a trauma has been experienced, children may begin to display restless or extreme behaviors. Some reactions might involve excessive anger, sadness, or withdrawal. Some children may start destroying toys, crying endlessly, or becoming detached from activities they had once enjoyed. Some young people might even appear to act like walking robots, showing no strong interest in anything or anybody. When children are exposed to trauma repeatedly, they may dissociate, creating a psychological distance between themselves and the arguments, abuse, or power plays going on around them. Others simply cut off their feelings, and still others begin to take an active role in the disruption, manipulating it to their advantage.

One of the most unfortunate outcomes is a child's loss of a sense of safety and security. The world stops being a place of wonder and amazement and starts to resemble a battleground where the child must take measures, often extreme measures, to find a place of refuge. These psychological wounds become evidence of "the world that hurt me," and children often avoid situations or persons that remind them of the trauma.

If the trauma includes sex, current research clearly shows that sexually abused children often have problems characterized by two clusters of symptoms:

- Negative feelings such as fear, worry, sadness, anger, isolation, shame, low self-worth, and lack of trust;
- disruptive behaviors such as aggression, inappropriate sexual activity, self-harm, and substance abuse.

Children with PTSD often will re-experience their traumatic experiences. They may have memories that repeat and replay themselves while they are awake or in their nightmares. They may feel that the trauma is recurring even if the context is quite different; a minor argument among peers may remind them of their perpetually dueling parents and they may overreact to the incident. Traumatized children may also express concern about death, complain about headaches or stomachaches, manifest anger outbursts, suffer from insomnia, and show an inability to concentrate. Those who engage in body cutting often state that this act brings a sense of relief from stress. Of course, this relief is temporary, because the stress is sure to return.

Children may also re-enact the traumatic experience using play—the primary language of childhood—often in conjunction with peers or with animals. They may engage in these re-enactments with peers, with pets, with dolls, or by themselves. As noted in Chapter 1, the symptoms of PTSD may last from a few months (acute PTSD) to many years (chronic PTSD).

## PTSD IN ADOLESCENCE

In adolescence, the manifestation of PTSD tends to be more like that seen among adults. The onset of PTSD in adolescence—a pivotal phase of human development—has a particularly damaging impact, since it may impair the acquisition of life skills needed to thrive and become independent in an "adult world." If these skills are not achieved before the onset of adulthood, the impairment can last a lifetime. Adolescence offers the beginnings of identity formation, cultivation of employment interests, and the bridging of childhood to adulthood, with the accompanying expression of sexual preference, relationship skills, and self-concept. PTSD can interfere with any of these developmental tasks.

One of the most serious consequences of PTSD during adolescence is its association with substance abuse. The use of alcohol and other drugs has immediate consequences in the form of increased accidents, injuries, and long-term effects in terms of occupational and familial instability and early mortality. Furthermore, substance abuse, in itself, is often a risk factor for additional traumatic exposures, either through accidents or interpersonal violence (Salter & Stallard, 2011).

Underlying these negative and destructive behaviors are the changes to a young person's brain following PTSD. We have already noted that children with symptoms of post-traumatic stress suffer poor function of the hippocampus, the brain structure that stores and retrieves memories. But another study found that a smaller hippocampus is itself a predisposing factor to PTSD (Orr et al., 2002). The brain does not distinguish between neurology and psychology or between cause and effect—and neither should practitioners working with young people who are PTSD survivors.

## FREQUENCY OF PTSD

What percent of the adolescent population develop PTSD? Studies have yielded varying results, depending on the part of the United States being examined and the age and economic level of the youngsters being studied. Much of what is currently known of the risk factors and consequences of PTSD among children and adolescents comes from case studies, often carried out on groups of young people who have experienced a shared trauma such as a natural disaster.

In one of these studies, the prevalence of PTSD in 384 adolescents in a Massachusetts community was examined. This investigation began when the participants were five years of age, and their lifetime prevalence of PTSD was determined by a standard set of interviews. The investigators found that 6 percent of the adolescents met full criteria for a PTSD diagnosis (Deykin, 1999).

A second longitudinal study involved 490 South Carolina adolescents. For this group, the lifetime occurrence of PTSD was 4 percent, with approximately 3 percent of females and 1 percent of males meeting the criteria for PTSD. A third study was a telephone survey of 4,023 adolescents indicating that the prevalence of PTSD was 8 percent. Despite some variation in the estimates in these three studies, it is apparent that the prevalence of PTSD among adolescents exceeds that found among adults in the 1980s. The occurrence of PTSD in these young populations probably reflects the well-documented increase of interpersonal violence in recent years (Deykin, 1999).

Differences in the prevalence of PTSD in the three groups surveyed are largely due to differences in the frequency of trauma exposure. For example, in the Massachusetts sample, 43 percent had experienced trauma, and 15 percent of the traumatized adolescents developed PTSD. In comparison, 16 percent of the South Carolina adolescents had experienced a qualifying trauma, but 21 percent of those suffered subsequent PTSD. Fewer members of the South Carolina group were traumatized, but those who suffered repeated traumas were more likely to develop PTSD. PTSD cannot occur among persons who have not experienced a trauma, so the frequency of trauma in a population is the major factor that determines the prevalence of PTSD.

As we mentioned earlier, not all persons who have suffered an event that qualifies as a trauma go on to develop PTSD. A number of other factors in addition to trauma influence the probability of developing PTSD. Among these factors are the characteristics of the trauma, the individual, the environment, and of the nature of support following the trauma. For example, interpersonal violence is a strong causative factor. In the Massachusetts study, rape was the event most likely to lead to PTSD. A different study of 297 adolescents receiving treatment for substance abuse also found that rape was the trauma most likely to cause PTSD. Although rape was far more common among the female subjects (40%), the few males who experienced rape (4%) had an almost identical risk of PTSD (77% vs. 75%) (Deykin, 1999).

Another study observed that rape victims may blame themselves for the abuse; if so, they resort more frequently to what is called *avoidance coping*. They try to sleep more than usual, avoid thinking about the problem, or resort to substance abuse. Self-blame is a form of *cognitive distortion*, which develops when young people do not understand why bad things have happened to them. Such personal myths as "Life should be fair" and "Nasty people should be punished" often are disrupted, leaving no alternative in their place (Deykin, 1999).

Apart from rape, other forms of assault, even if only witnessed, can be activating factors in PTSD. In one study, children who had witnessed domestic violence, although they themselves were not victims, showed significantly more PTSD symptoms than children who had not witnessed such violence. The marked difference in the two groups may have been due to the fact that the aggressor was frequently the father, thus dividing the child's loyalty and producing stress that was difficult, if not impossible, to manage. But the effects of interpersonal violence are not limited to the victims; the perpetrators may suffer as well. When imprisoned juvenile delinquents were studied, one out of three met criteria for PTSD, and for many of them, the symptoms of PTSD resulted from violence they had perpetrated on others (Deykin, 1999).

Research on the consequences of natural disasters and accidents suggests that, in the initial phase, there can be considerable trauma-related symptoms, but the effects tend to diminish faster than in the case of interpersonal violence. When a dam burst in Buffalo Creek, West Virginia in 1972, many people were killed and considerable property was destroyed. One out of three of the survivors demonstrated PTSD, but 17 years later only 7 percent still had PTSD symptoms. In contrast, PTSD due to trauma unrelated to the flood decreased only from 6 percent to 4 percent (Deykin, 1999).

In a study of 5,687 children and adolescents who had experienced Hurricane Hugo in 1989, about 5 percent had symptoms sufficiently severe to be classified as PTSD. The investigators stated that younger children and females of any age reported more symptoms. Males reported symptoms focused on poor memory and concentration, while females reported symptoms involved repetitive thoughts of the hurricane, as well as emotional numbing and social isolation (Deykin, 1999).

Youth whose houses were damaged, who became displaced, or whose parents lost employment as a result of the hurricane were twice as likely to meet criteria for PTSD as those who did not experience such events. However, the most important predictive factor was the level of a young person's anxiety and emotional reactivity during the storm, suggesting that the basic emotional makeup of the children and teens studied played an important role in the development of PTSD. We would, therefore, consider emotional makeup a *predisposing* factor, and the hurricane itself an *activating* factor in PTSD.

Youth who were able to remain with their families were less vulnerable to PTSD, regardless of property damage. The importance of a supportive family in lessening the effects of natural disasters, accidents, and even war is a common theme that emerges from most of these research studies. When 103 Israeli children who were residents of kibbutzim communities that frequently received enemy shelling were compared with 90 children who lived in kibbutzim that had never been shelled, there were no major differences. The children less likely to develop PTSD symptoms had experienced more family and community support. These children experienced the shelling not as individuals, but as members of a cohesive group that provided closeness, affiliation, and mutual support (Balaban, 2009; Salter & Stallard, 2011).

## TREATMENT

The best approach to child and adolescent trauma is prevention. The better informed parents, teachers, or social groups are about PTSD, the more likely it is that they will take steps to prevent young people from being traumatized. However, once the trauma has occurred, early intervention is essential; support from parents, teachers, and peers is important. Emphasis needs to be placed on establishing a feeling of safety for children who have survived a motor vehicle accident, a physical assault, or the death of a loved one. While the majority of children involved in potentially traumatizing events appear to cope reasonably well, there is a need to develop a better understanding of protective and resilience factors, such as family support and positive attitudes that decrease the potential negative effects of the event. It is also important to remember that young people may suffer from many stress disorders, not all of them severe enough to be classified as PTSD. But a child or a teen who may not meet the full criteria for PTSD can still experience difficulties in functioning on a day-by-day basis.

Early intervention appears to show promise once a potentially traumatizing event has occurred. "Acute intervention" is a term used to describe treatment provided in the first six weeks after the event. A novel approach of acute intervention implemented in a Connecticut community helped improve communication between children who had experienced stress and their parents or other caregivers. The Child and Family Traumatic Stress Intervention (CHTSI) taught 106 young people between the ages of 7 and 17 to recognize and manage traumatic stress symptoms within one month of a potentially traumatizing event. Children were referred by police, a forensic sexual abuse program, or the local pediatric emergency department (Berkowitz, Stover, & Marans, 2011).

The CFTSI intervention began with an assessment of the young person's trauma history and a preliminary visit with the parent or other caregiver, focusing on their essential role in the process. Within the first two sessions, there were activities to help improve communication between the young person and the caregiver, as well as other measures that helped give the child or teen the feeling of support. At the end of each of the next two sessions, the clinician, caregiver, and child together decided on a homework assignment to practice coping skills. During all four sessions, the young people were taught behavioral skills to help them recognize and manage symptoms of traumatic stress.

In follow-up studies, the CFTSI intervention was able to prevent PTSD in three out of four children who had been exposed to a potentially traumatizing event such as bullying at school or family violence. A more conventional treatment used with a similar number of children did not attain the same degree of success as did CFTSI in reducing sleep disturbances, emotional numbness, angry outbursts, or difficulties concentrating. The authors of the study claimed that this was the first report of a preventive intervention to improve outcomes in children who had experienced a potentially traumatizing event, and the first to reduce the onset of PTSD in children.

Psychotherapy and counseling at the individual, group, or family level usually allow the child to speak, draw, play, or write about the event. Susan Clancy (2010) maintains that it empowers young PTSD survivors to tell their own stories. *Trauma-Focused Cognitive-Behavior Therapy* and such psychodynamic treatments as *Child-Parent Psychotherapy* may help PTSD survivors to reduce their stress, fears, and worries. Other strategies include psychoeducation to correct cognitive distortions, grief counseling if a loved one has died, and therapeutic massage, administered by a trained practitioner.

*Expressive Arts Therapies* are structured to allow for a safe, non-threatening space for the young person to explore and master elements of the trauma. Many of these practitioners note that traumatic material is "stored" in the brain's right hemisphere (except in the case of some left-handed people). This is the same part of the cerebral cortex that is highly active during painting, dancing, sculpting, and other modalities used by art therapists. Traumatic material, when recalled, is typically expressed in visual—not verbal—form, giving an edge to expressive arts therapies over talk therapies, especially with children. The goal of sand play, finger painting, expressive movement, and similar techniques is emotional regulation, with the creative process serving to attain this goal. Expressive Art Therapies can be used in conjunction with cognitive-behavior therapy, psychodynamic therapy, and other forms of treatment.

Medication may be useful to deal with agitation, anxiety, or depression (Donnelly, 2009). It can be supplemented with teaching children relaxation exercises, helping them to construct a cohesive story about the traumatic event, and assisting them to learn to cope with reminders of the trauma. PTSD survivors are more likely to thrive if they can regain optimism, positive expectancies, self-confidence, and a sense of direction for their lives. With the sensitivity and support of families and health care workers, children and teens with PTSD can learn to cope with their memories of the trauma and go on to lead healthy and productive lives.

The effective elements of these interventions need to be assessed. It is especially important to examine the effectiveness of brief early interventions to see which of these are most successful in reducing symptoms and preventing chronic PTSD. The education of parents and other caregivers is an essential part of treating young PTSD survivors. Whereas parents may misinterpret a child's "acting out" as retaliation for his or her condition, it is more likely to represent an overload of the brain's normal mechanism for handling fear, shame, and other emotions that typically accompany PTSD.

In fact, advances in neurology may make it possible for traumatic memories to be "erased" from the brain or at least reduced in their intensity. Identifying the precise neurons that constitute a *memory trace* is challenging, because they are distributed in many areas. However, laboratory work with neurons in the amygdala that are activated by fear memory expression has shown some promise (Han et al., 2009). PTSD involves fear memories that simply refuse to disappear;

perhaps neurochemicals can be developed in the future that will send them on their way.

We will close this chapter by describing two instances of trauma, one from Canada and one from the Philippines. We already mentioned that PTSD does not play politics; either does it conform to any particular national boundary.

## DAVID'S HISTORY OF TRAUMA

We have presented several case studies where PTSD was accompanied by such emotions as fear and anxiety. However, shame plays an important part as well, especially when one's reputation and self-concept are threatened by the traumatizing event (Budden, 2009). All of these emotions played out in the case of David, whose Native American name was Copper Seal.

In 1894, St. Michael's Residential School for Boys was established in Alert Bay, British Columbia. All the students were Native Americans, and the stated goal of the school was to prepare them for entry into mainstream Canadian society. In 1972, David, who was six years of age at the time, was among those taken from his family and enrolled in St. Michael's. This act was condoned by Canadian law, and parental permission was not required. The separation from his family was the first of several traumatizing events that led to David's chronic PTSD.

After crying all night in the dormitory, David attended his first class the following day. St. Michael's was a church-related school, but followed a nationwide curriculum for Native Americans, as did all the parochial schools, whether they were Protestant or Roman Catholic, and whether they served boys or girls. In addition to academic courses, there were classes in carpentry, furniture building, and farming, and animal husbandry (the care of livestock). There were no classes in fishing, despite the fact that this was the primary way that David's family and neighbors on Inlet Bay earned their living.

On the second day of class, David was called to an instructor's private office and told that he had to be taught "discipline." The instructor locked the door and proceeded to sodomize the young boy. David returned to his classroom, bleeding from the rectum. His teacher scolded him and made him clean up his seat and desk before he could leave for the day. The sexual abuse left David with a feeling of shame, as it violated his self-concept of active masculinity, substituting an image of a passive boy playing a female role. In addition, social shame resulted from his treatment by the classroom teacher, as everyone in the class could guess why David was bleeding.

When David's class was allowed home visits, he immediately told his parents about the abuse. His father cut him short, saying, "We don't talk about such things in this family" while his mother remained silent. David returned to

St. Michael's and spent the next eight years being sexually abused by both male and female instructors, both laypersons and members of the clergy. Female instructors were especially fond of ordering two or more boys to abuse each other sexually while they watched and sometimes laughed. In the meantime, David was grimacing in pain and holding back his anger.

Once David was able to leave St. Michael's, he entered a public school. By that time his PTSD was accompanied by flashbacks and nightmares. The public school lacked the rigid control of the parochial school, and David's pent-up anger exploded, fueled by the shame he felt. He directed his hostility against his classmates, his teachers, school property, and even against himself. He entered the world of illegal drugs and stole money to obtain them. He became an example of co-morbidity; that is, his chronic PTSD went hand-in-hand with cocaine addiction and, eventually, alcoholism.

David began to sell illegal drugs and ended up in jail. In contrast to St. Michael's, David found imprisonment rather pleasant. He worked very hard in prison, but it was not as exhausting as the farm work he was forced to do in the residential school. His fellow prisoners did not make fun of him, as most of them had longer histories of criminal activity than did David. Further, David was assured of three meals a day and a better menu than that offered at St. Michael's, where he was perpetually hungry. Even the beds were more comfortable in prison.

In 1991, a Native American survivor of St. Michael's sued the school. It had taken all that while for someone to gain access to the legal system and to bypass the social shame that had kept others from taking similar action. In 1999, St. Michael's was closed, and the Canadian government set aside two billion Canadian dollars to reimburse boys and girls, now young men and women, who could demonstrate that they had been abused. Indeed, the government organized several "levels of abuse," and David's experience qualified him for a handsome financial settlement.

David took back his Indian name, Copper Seal, which St. Michael's had forbidden him to use. He bought a fishing boat with the compensation money and began to earn an honest living selling flounder, salmon, and other fish that he caught. He began to date a young woman, Meg. Although not a PTSD survivor herself, Meg was attentive when David told her his story of eight years of abuse, shame, and anger.

David avoided anything having to do with Christianity, but found spiritual comfort and inspiration in the sacred ceremonies, songs, and dances of his Northwest Coast Indian tribe. Ironically, these were the same ceremonies that his instructors at St. Michael's had deemed "pagan," "uncivilized," and the "work of the devil." David Copper Seal reflected, "I have seen civilization up close, and if St. Michael's was an example of it, I would prefer to be a pagan."

## FLORA'S HISTORY OF TRAUMA

Here is another report, as portrayed in another trauma survivor's own words.

Hi. My name is Flora Mae Lozano, I live in the Philippines, and I am 19 years old. Well, most people know that life can sometimes hit rock bottom before it gets better. My life is a prime example of this. I am writing this because I have friends whose problems, although tiny for me, are big for them. I think my experiences may help others. Are you ready? Sit tight! Here goes!

I was born on the 31st of July to a happy, loving family. Mom and dad were always there so I never came from a "broken family." Life was always happy and fun until I became 8 years of age.

Every weekend Mom would take me, my sister Karen, and my brother Darren to see my Granddad. How could he not be trusted? Mom saw no reason to be suspicious. So, sure enough, we were left there for him to babysit us. But a week after my 8th birthday, my Granddad became more than a babysitter.

About 15 minutes after Mom left us with Granddad, we were allowed to play outside in the garden as it was summer at the time. Suddenly I was told that I had done something wrong. To this day I still don't know what I did that deserved what happened to me. In any case my Granddad sent me indoors and told me to sit on the sofa. Then he sat next to me. Granddad told me that I had to put my hand somewhere, and he would show me where. Of course that "somewhere" was inside of his trousers. I was too young to realize what was happening so I went ahead and did it.

Granddad then told me that my punishment was over and this was a secret. I should not tell Mom, otherwise she would be mad at what I had done and that I would bring shame to my family. Numb to what had happened, I was allowed to go back into the garden and play with my brother and sister. Later, Mom collected us and Granddad was playing it cool. I did not tell my Mom and in some ways I blame myself for not telling her or someone else.

About four months later, Mom left my sister and me with Granddad again. The three of us were in the living room and I was told I had been a very bad girl and that I had to go into the kitchen and wait for my punishment. I was made to perform sexual acts on my Granddad, and he touched me all over my body. I started to put up a fight but then I just became numb and I let him do it. I was told again that Mom was not to know. If I did tell Mom and Dad, they would be angry and then Granddad would hurt me something terrible.

This continued on and off for about a year. When I was 9, I decided to stop it. I screamed out but he covered my mouth. I was told that I had done terrible things and he then proceeded to rape me. I still wonder why Mom never noticed the abuse because I sustained bruises all over my body because of how violent he had been. Again, Granddad told me he'd kill me if I told Mom. Scared to death I told no one, keeping up the happy-go-lucky-child I pretended to be on the outside. But inside I really suffered.

Throughout the next two years this occurred quite regularly. I was raped at least two dozen times. When I was 11 I begged Mom not to take me to see Granddad anymore and after begging constantly she finally agreed. I felt that this was freedom at last! Now I am just finishing college and I have only just told Mom about the experiences. They have stayed in my own mind even though I hoped that the memories would go away. My flashbacks have been coming back regularly and I still don't know how to deal with them. But one thing I knew is that I had to tell the police. So two days before my 16th birthday I reported it. And then I found out that there were other members in my family he had abused, but not as bad as me. He abused both my sister and my brother, and none of us ever dared discuss it because of his threats and because of our shame.

I often get suicidal thoughts and have tried to kill myself a few times. What happened to Granddad? Well I am still going through the courts for justice and he has been charged on four different counts. I have to go to court and give evidence. Needless to say I am scared stiff.

Now I am 19. Two years ago I was diagnosed with Irritable Bowel Disorder and Crohn's Disease. After months of being in and out of hospitals, I am controlling it by venting my feelings and occasionally using painkillers. I do suffer from depression now and again, but I am studying to be a midwife and I am far happier then I have ever been. I have started to learn how to love myself, look after myself, and most of all to take care of my own needs. Once my Granddad is punished, it will bring some sort of closure to that whole part of my life and I think my physical ailments will start to clear up. In fact, my flashbacks have already decreased.

I have a new boyfriend who loves me and protects me. But I know inside there is no way anyone could have loved me until—and here's the bottom line—I started to love myself. One thing I know for sure is that life is too short to live in the past and I am surviving. Are you?

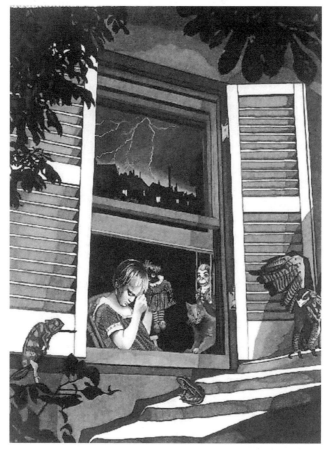

The Storm Child (Reproduced from the original art of Dierdre Luzwick.)

# 5

# Four Cases of PTSD

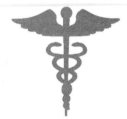

S o far, we have provided a review of the diverse terrain of PTSD from both diagnostic and historical perspectives. Now, we need to discuss how PTSD can present itself by describing several traumatic experiences. Trauma does not discriminate; it can affect anyone susceptible to its nature. We only know its face by the way it expresses itself. How do we know? We know by observing the individual's behavior, attitudes, and language—both verbal and non-verbal. We know by seeing how that individual relates—or does not relate—to other people. We know by listening to what these individuals have to say about themselves, in other words, how they describe their life stories.

We are never sure who will become traumatized due to life's many stressors. About half of all Americans undergo terrifying, frightening incidents throughout their lives, but only about one in ten develop PTSD as a result. To illustrate this, we will review some cases of individuals who experienced traumatizing events that led to PTSD diagnoses, and depict the complexity of their symptoms. This procedure will help cultivate an appreciation of the intricacies of trauma and its various expressions.

Remember that there are three major clusters of symptoms that aid diagnosis: (1) re-experiencing the trauma in nightmares and intrusive flashbacks, (2) emotional numbing and avoidance of social interactions, and (3) behaviors associated with hyperarousal. The latter group of symptoms can range from losing one's temper to finding it difficult to concentrate. Now, we will present the stories of four individuals who have been diagnosed as having PTSD followed by a discussion of how each of them displayed the three major clusters of symptoms.

## CASE ONE: THE VETERAN

We begin by revisiting Daryl Paulson's reflections on his life once his service in Vietnam came to an end. Paulson wrote:

> For those of us who survived the "Nam," our day to leave the country finally came. We were going back to the WORLD—a name we gave to the United States—home to round-eyed, friendly, and affectionate women, home to a world where the streets were asphalt-paved and there were flush toilets, hot and cold running water, food other than C-rations, and plenty of cold beer.
>
> Unlike the mythological hero who—after going through the initiatory ordeal to find the Golden Fleece or the Holy Grail—brings back his trophy to share with all, the Vietnam veteran brought back no treasure. That is, he attained no positive knowledge or treasure that he could share with the others in his community. When our 707 landed at El Toro Marine Air Station, which had been deactivated, I was secretly preparing for a hero's welcome. I think all of us reasoned that we would get a doubly strong welcome because we had fought in spite of the absence of any explicit government plan to win the war. For example, Congress and/or the president would decide to bomb North Vietnam one week, but stop bombing the next. This on-again, off-again strategy was terrible for our morale. We would often wonder, *Why the hell are we here if our leaders cannot make up their minds whether to fight the war or bail out?* Given these unusually hard conditions, we now thought we would be rewarded.
>
> We landed and walked out of the plane to our homecoming reception. I saw *three* people waiting for us. That was it! They were Marine wives who had volunteered to serve cookies and Kool-Aid to us. Where was everyone else? Where were the women to welcome us home? They should be here, I thought.
>
> Once in the air terminal, we were escorted to waiting military buses and driven to Camp Pendleton Marine Base for discharge or reassignment. During the drive, some college-age people screamed obscenities at us and flipped us the bird. I can still remember their yelling something about our being "warmongers."
>
> At Camp Pendleton we were swiftly processed and bused to Los Angeles International Airport to schedule flights home. At the Los Angeles airport, I went to a bar to have a couple of drinks while waiting for my flight. This was an especially big event for me. It was my first legal drink in the United States and in a bar, for now I was of age, 21. I felt like being friendly, so I tried to start a conversation with two women sitting next to me, but they ignored me. Then I tried to talk to a couple of guys, but they, too, ignored me. It began to dawn on me that no one cared that I had served in the Vietnam War. I felt like a misfit.

The lack of care and concern for what I had been through was even apparent with my friends when I arrived home and went out drinking with them. Things were different. I noticed not only that they did not care about the war, but that I was now different from these guys. They were caught up in being "cool" and contriving to attract women. I just did not care. I had just seen hundreds of U.S. servicemen killed; I had also seen hundreds and hundreds of North Vietnamese soldiers killed and had tried to kill as many of them as I could. I had faced thirteen months of not knowing if I would die that day. Now, to worry about my hair or a woman seemed petty and meaningless. To protect myself from the meaninglessness of this life, I found a friend that night. It was a friend who would keep me calm and mellow for the next two years. That friend was beer.

The first several weeks back in the states were also hard on me when I had to describe the Vietnam experience to my friends. After a friend asked me, I thought to myself, *How could I describe that hell in words?* I felt anger, frustration, fear, and hate, all welling up inside of me. I felt like beating the table in utter frustration, but instead I calmly took another drink of beer, said, "It was real bad," and left it at that. But I knew—not only consciously, but in the center of my being—that something was terribly and painfully wounded within me. My friend did not really care. He was more interested in collecting information to support his anti-war beliefs. For me, however, it was different. He had opened up a huge wound inside me. I recalled the friends from my unit whom I saw killed—John O., John B., Jose, Peter, Jocko, Fraizer, Rocko, Pork Chops, and Glen. What had they died for? They died for nothing—nothing but bullshit. I took another drink of beer . . . and another . . . and another.

I think all of us veterans shared a sense of condemnation. We felt a kind of deep guilt that sent terror to the very core of our being. If we had been wrong about the war, were we not similar to Nazi criminals? Was there really a reason to keep on living? How could we live with ourselves, having seen and experienced all the brutalities of war and survived it, only to realize that our involvement served no positive purpose? I sensed the overt damage within myself. I remember fantasizing about how warm and caring I would be when I got back from Vietnam. I would find that special woman and devote my life to our relationship. The entire time I was in Vietnam, I thought to myself how nice it would be to be held by a warm, loving woman, to watch her laugh and smile as I teased her. I would fantasize over and over what it would be like.

When I did return, things were different. I found that I did not really like to be with women; they made me nervous. To be held by a woman made me feel very vulnerable. Instead of feeling good, I would feel terribly sad and afraid in her arms. It was almost like being a little boy again, in need of a mother to hug away my pain. But I was 21 years old; I was too old to need a mother figure. Since these vulnerable feelings were, I thought, a sign of my weak character, I began avoiding any closeness with women.

I did find that I could get close to a woman when I drank. Drinking made relationships with women much easier; I did not feel vulnerable and could use them for sexual gratification. After all, what was a woman for, except to fuck? Many other veterans I talked with shared this experience. In fact, our new motto became, "Find them, feel them, fuck them, and forget them." We had to distance ourselves from any meaningful encounter with women because we felt that we could not share with them what we had experienced. How could you tell your girlfriend what it was like for you to shoot another human being? How could you tell her how vulnerable and scared you had felt, never knowing if you would live another hour the whole time you were in Vietnam? How could you tell her what it was like to kick dead enemy soldiers because you were so angry at them for killing your friends? I was afraid to tell any woman what it was like.

How could I tell her about the horror I felt watching a dump truck taking the corpses of seventeen of my friends to be embalmed? How could I tell her what I felt when I watched their blood drip and flow from the tailgate onto the ground? How could I tell her how deeply I hurt, of the agony I was in, and how gnawing my suffering was? How could I tell her that the pain and guilt followed me like a beast tracking its prey? How could I tell her that the pain hounded me at night, during the day, and even while making love? What would she think of me if I told her? I feared that if any woman knew this about me, she would freak out, go into convulsions, vomit, and totally reject me for being such a disgusting human being.

What was I to do? I did what seemed best: I drank and drank and drank. So did most of the other veterans I knew, and since we drank so much and so often—while pretending it was partying—it was hard for others to recognize it as a way of masking our own pain. But God, it was there.

Then one day, it happened. I had an anxiety attack. I was sitting in an accounting class when I suddenly felt as though I were dying. My heart began to pound; I was becoming dizzy and my eyes would not focus. I began gasping for breath and sweating profusely. I began to "freak out." I walked out of class, pretending everything was okay, and went immediately to the student health service. There, however, the doctor who examined me could find nothing wrong with me. To me, this meant that something very serious was wrong with me. I began to relive feelings of being near death, as I had been in Vietnam. This totally confused me.

After suffering about five more panic attacks and running to the doctor, he sent me to a psychiatrist. I did not relish the idea of having mental problems, but I needed to be spared from this new form of suffering. When I saw the psychiatrist, he disinterestedly asked me what my symptoms were. I told him, and he prescribed two kinds of tranquilizers, as well as an antidepressant, and told me to take it easy. That was the last thing I could think of doing, I was so distraught with my life. I tried, though. I tried to enjoy target shooting with my .22 rifle, but I began to physically shake so badly while aiming, I could not shoot. Shooting had been my favorite pastime, and now it was gone. I just could not endure it; it made me too tense.

No fear impacted me as much as the fear I felt during thunder storms. Even though I knew thunder was caused by lightning, the sound of thunder would send me right back to Vietnam. It felt as if I were undergoing a rocket attack. I would have to drop to the ground to protect myself from incoming. (Paulson & Krippner, 2007, pp. 166–174)

## CASE TWO: THE COLLEGE STUDENT

Sarah was an ambitious and above-average student throughout her high school career in a small town in Iowa. She discovered that the relationships with her friends, family, and her boyfriend were of great importance, inspiring her to express care for them in gifts, affection, and listening. Sarah would often volunteer her time at human service organizations to both help others and cultivate her own interests and inspirations for future work. Nothing would block her from achieving her goals! After graduation, Sarah prepared for her upcoming collegiate journey to a nearby university. Full of excitement and passion for learning, she could not wait to begin. Though touched with sadness at being at a distance from her loved ones, she would often write letters and call her boyfriend to soothe the time away from him.

It was not a surprise to Sarah that she immediately found great excitement in attending her psychology courses. Texts and theories on learning, emotions, and memory captivated her. She would often spend hours in the library poring over studies and new developments in the field. But one evening forever altered Sarah's philosophy of human nature and psychology, but it did not come from a textbook or journal article.

Winters were harsh on her campus, especially with the library being located far from her dorm, what amounted to a half-mile walk or an average of five city blocks. Leaving just before the library closed in the late evening, Sarah departed in a rush in order to let her forgetful roommate back into their room. Yes, her roommate had left her key behind again and reached Sarah by cell phone to tell her to hurry back. As Sarah neared the unlit path between the tennis courts, the darkness came alive with a bulky figure that soon rendered her powerless.

Although Sarah struggled, she could not escape. The force was much stronger than anything she could muster, and with his hand over her mouth and his knife near her throat, the power to survive without resistance took hold as the rape commenced. Once her assailant left the scene, Sarah lay helpless on the ground in a timeless space of pain, horror, and fear.

Sarah's soul was wounded. She could not cry, she could not feel, she felt lost and voiceless. Her strength and her very identity felt shattered. Sarah's sense of trust departed that night, leaving her adrift in a now dangerous world of terror and helplessness. Her grades suffered as did her relationships, including that with her boyfriend. They lost all meaning.

Sarah was not able to communicate her difficult daily experiences, let alone share the story of that night, nor could she relate to others as she once did. Rather, Sarah became haunted by shadows, often seeing her attacker in darkness and in nightmares. Sarah was too frightened to leave her room at night and even found excuses to stay there during the day. Hiding from the world around her, Sarah felt safe only in her room, even though she barely spoke to her roommate. And at night even her room was not safe because her attacker returned in her nightmares to repeat his violation.

## CASE THREE: THE EMERGENCY RESPONSE WORKER

Michael fought for the lives of his patients. No matter how difficult the situation, he committed himself to the welfare of each person he was serving. After 15 years as an emergency medical technician or EMT in upstate New York, he felt a great sense of pride at being able to help so many people. He had seen and done it all—extracting people mangled in car accidents, arriving at the locations of both "successful" and "unsuccessful" suicides, attending to severely burned victims, and caring for numerous individuals suffering from a myriad of natural and human-made catastrophes.

But despite his passion and his ability to be of service, Michael began to notice some changes in his personality. The excitement he felt when he went to work and to help started to diminish. Sometimes Michael found himself calling in sick, when previously he had taken only one sick day in the past two years. Therefore, Michael decided to take some time off and "recharge his batteries," but his batteries did not recharge. Despite his best efforts, Michael began to notice that he was losing his "edge." He was often awakened by graphic and horrifying nightmares of his patients, glimpsing their images during the day as well. He was becoming more agitated, was not sleeping well, and was easily "set-off" at work and around others. Eventually, he began disconnecting himself from his colleagues, friends, and family.

Michael was engaged in an internal struggle, finding some brief solace in his nightly ritual drinking, often to the point of intoxication. Alcohol helped reduce his anxiety and allowed him to fall asleep, but often, sound slumber could not be found. He would awaken from a nightmare and then was too agitated to fall back to sleep. Michael fought to reclaim himself, but could not find solid ground. He had become overtaken by his haunting memories, frequent agitation, and daily torment.

## CASE FOUR: THE CAR ACCIDENT SURVIVOR

It had been two months since her car accident at the intersection in a large city in Illinois. Teesha's memory kept bringing her to the event as if it had just happened minutes ago. On her way home from work one rainy night, a drunk driver in a minivan ran a red light and hit Teesha's Honda Civic. Thankfully,

Teesha was not injured, at least not physically. However, ever since the accident, she had not been able to leave her home. Rather, she was terrorized by intense flashbacks of the accident. These often occurred whenever she attempted to go outside. She found herself lost in a life of terror and unpredictability governed by a daily anxiety that consumed her every thought, movement, and breath. Teesha's daily routine was not charted by pleasant activity and productive work. Instead it was governed by avoiding all possible reminders of the event, especially outside where cars lurk like dangerous monsters.

Teesha used to exercise daily, engage in outside activities, and spend her time working, shopping, or going places to visit close friends and family. Eventually, Teesha lost her corporate job of 10 years and began working from home, sending mailers and living on a low, but sustainable income. After one month, she decided to regain some vestige of her former routine. She made a telephone call to initiate a gym membership, but quickly cancelled her subscription that same day, feeling nauseous and dizzy when she tried to go out of the door.

Not giving much thought to the aborted gym experience, Teesha began looking for work again. A number of agencies and businesses caught her interest, so she prepared resumes, faxed the appropriate paperwork, and scheduled interviews. However, everything changed as she began driving to her appointments. As was the case with her earlier experience enrolling at the gym, Teesha endured panic, nausea, psychological paralysis, and an overwhelming sense of helplessness.

Teesha could no longer stand to be near family members or people in her community. She struggled with how embarrassed she felt when she made up excuses to leave their presence early or to avoid them altogether. Teesha felt discomfort most of the time, and found that she was easily irritable. She had difficulty sleeping, and became angry when she could not control—much less subdue—her feelings and reactions.

Teesha eventually lost contact with her friends and withdrew from any attempt toward building any intimate connection or relationship with others. Her life interests and passions dissolved into a passive sea of boredom.

### Evaluation of the Cases

As we can see, there is no "one size fits all" lens to apply to someone's experiences so as to allow for a typical case of PTSD. What then, are the common psychological and social expressions or symptoms for someone experiencing post-traumatic stress disorder? Even trained psychotherapists cannot speak for another's experience for they are not the ones who are doing the experiencing. However, they can observe and listen to the individual recall his or her torment, anguish, and distress. Let's consider the above case examples and provide an in-depth review, extrapolating each of the major PTSD criteria in an attempt to better appreciate and highlight the ways that PTSD symptoms might be expressed.

## INTRUSION AND RE-EXPERIENCING

Let's imagine for a moment that you are in a space where you feel safe and comfortable. You feel that you can do anything in this space—it is yours. Now, imagine that someone has unexpectedly entered your space, uninvited and unwelcome. This person just barged in, disregarding your privacy. This is an intrusion, a forceful invasion and violation.

Now, you have some idea of PTSD's most prominent feature. It is the *experience* of an event that makes it traumatic. That terrifying, shattering, devastating intrusive experience then repeats itself in your imagination. As a result, it continues to intrude upon experiences that used to be enjoyable and comfortable. Daryl Paulson's combat experiences and inability to reintegrate into society began to erode his ability to function and rebuild his life as a civilian. Intrusion took the form of being "haunted by faces" in flashbacks and nightmares, tormented by social rejection, and recurring feelings of despair. Marie was plagued by nightmares in which she would re-experience the rape. During the day she would have intrusive thoughts of being harmed if she ventured outside. Michael's intensive exposure to wounded men and women began to trouble him, largely through flashbacks of his experiences. Teesha's car accident invaded her thoughts; she re-experienced that event and could not resume her previous way of living.

No matter what any of these people tried to do, their memories did not remain in their cabinet of past memories, but continued to linger in the halls of daily living, stealing any chance for them to move easily through life. Each of these person's experiencing was unique to them, although the end result was the same—continual torment and a violation of their functioning, blocking any attempts to merge the past into the present.

## AVOIDANCE AND EMOTIONAL NUMBING

Though the term "avoidance" may seem obvious in definition, the myriad of forms it can take are not so apparent. When a person exhibits avoidance behavior, he or she attempts to keep away from, escape from, or shun elements associated with the traumatizing event. Some of these reminders can include similar locations, sounds, smells, and any other particular trigger connected to elements of the trauma.

Individuals affected by PTSD undertake everything they can muster to protect themselves from allowing a trauma to occur again. These attempts often appear as extreme and bizarre behaviors, as was the case with the individuals we profiled. Daryl used alcohol and disconnected himself from social relationships. Marie could not connect to those once close to her and was unable to feel any type of pleasure in life, a condition technically called *anhedonia*. Michael also avoided others and often drank himself to sleep. Teesha felt she had to stay home in order to find a sense of safety; she made up excuses that circumvented ever going outside. All four were emotionally numb much of the time; it was as if their feelings had been siphoned from their psyches, or as if their souls had been damaged or lost.

The principal impact that social avoidance has in all of these cases is internal. External cues or triggers remind people of the traumatizing event, and so to avoid discomfort the individual attempts to avoid anything similar. But there are numerous reminders of the traumatic experience, so it is inevitable that inappropriate and harmful responses will be made no matter how similar the context is to the original incident. No matter what each of our four men and women did to reduce the anxiety of their experiences, they still were thrown back on themselves—always with the vivid memory of what happened to produce stress so severe that it could not be assimilated or managed.

If one's personal identity is not restored following the trauma, their efforts to avoid the intrusive and insidious nature of trauma will be ineffective in providing any long-term relief. As many tribal shamans and other native healers observe, their very soul has been lost, the casualty of an event that overwhelmed their capacity to maintain the balance they need to proceed on life's journey.

### Hyperarousal

Intense anxiety is the core agent behind arousal responses that exceed ordinary reactions to life's stresses and hassles. There are inevitable bumps in one's journey through life, and for PTSD survivors, these trigger a reminder of the traumatizing event. This memory typically evokes a response known as hyperarousal, most often a heightened state of anxiety. All of us feel anxious once in a while, but in PTSD the anxiety is more severe and longer-lasting, the reaction to a trigger is extreme and exaggerated. This reaction could take the form of irritability, a shock or startle, a lack of concentration, a sleep disorder, or an extreme sensitivity to surprises or shifts in one's daily routine.

For example, in combat, it is common for soldiers to hear loud noises as the result of the firing of rounds of ammunition, the launching of missiles, the exploding of improvised explosive devices (IEDs), and the strafing from tank warfare or airplanes. However, these events are not common in most cultural settings outside of warfare. So when veterans return to their ordinary settings and begin to overreact to the slamming of a door, the backfiring of a car, or the setting off of a firecracker, this is actually a *normal reaction* for them. It is also normal when a traumatized combat veteran returns to a non-combat zone, such as his or her home, and reacts intensely to such noise events. The veteran may hide, drop to the floor, or become agitated. This is what psychologists call a "conditioned response" which is a reaction, once entrenched, that will occur even when the stimulus is somewhat different and the outcome harmless instead of life-threatening.

In each of the cases we discussed above, there are similar instances of hyperarousal, but each was unique to the individual. In all of our case scenarios, agitation, startle responses, and sleep problems plagued the life experiences of the men and women with PTSD diagnoses. However, their hyperaroused reactions were not understood as normal reactions, either by the person who had been traumatized or by their family and friends. Instead, the reaction was seen as awkward at best and as alarming or even dangerous at worse. These reactions from friends and family members often slowed down the PTSD survivor's assimilation of the experience. Nobody was around to help these survivors accept these behaviors as being normal reactions to abnormal events. So not only was the original event traumatizing, but the personal and social reactions served to maintain the trauma. The consequences led to behaviors that were considered to be "abnormal," the avoidance of social contact being but one of them.

As we noted before, such words as "crazy" and "mentally ill" are social constructs. The PTSD survivor is judged to display "symptoms" that are "pathological" and to manifest conditions that amount to a "disorder." In 2011, U.S. Army General Peter Chiarelli advocated using the term "post-traumatic stress," dropping the word "disorder," arguing that the latter term unnecessarily stigmatizes veterans' natural responses to the emotional and violent experiences of battle. General Chiarelli made an excellent point, one that is in agreement with our contention that these reactions are natural and normal reactions to situations that are unnatural and abnormal. It is warfare, rape, bullying, and torture that deserve the label "abnormal," not the person who has survived these unnatural events.

## WHERE DO THEY GO FROM HERE?

### Attachment and Intimacy

One social construct commonly used in psychology is "attachment." What does it mean to "attach"? For our purposes, it refers to the bond, or connection that can be formed between oneself and others. Sometimes people may have a positive bond with others, where they cultivate closeness; at other times they may have a negative bond, where they endorse distance, avoiding certain relationships. The four cases we discussed all demonstrated severe problems with attachment following their traumas.

John Bowlby (1988), a pioneering psychotherapist who helped develop what is called *attachment theory*, premised that individuals develop what he called "internal working models" of how they will relate to the world around them and to others in that world. This model is cultivated in infancy, primarily through the way that parents and other caregivers relate to a child. The relating styles of the caregivers are based on those individuals' sense of self-worth and lovability. These models, in turn, affect the infant's perception of the caregiver's trustworthiness and dependability. These perceptions set the pattern for how the infant, when a child or adolescent, will relate to other people.

Bowlby conjectured that a person's internal working models will serve as relatively enduring templates or reference points for his or her subsequent intimate adult relationships. Bowlby further argued that any shortcomings in these ways of relating are most likely triggered when one is stressed, fatigued, or ill. All of these are internal states that activate and determine whether one pursues what Bowlby referred to as "proximity seeking" or "proximity avoidance." The former term refers to a need for closeness while the latter refers to a desire for distance (Lopez, Melendez, Sauer, Berger, & Wyssmann, 1998, p. 80).

In other words, the experiences we have with people early in our lives help determine how we attach to others, either positively or negatively, either gravitating toward intimate connections or holding others at a distance. What can we learn from all this information about attachment theory? Well, we can understand that we are relational beings by nature. Relationships shape our ability to navigate through life. The language, emotions, and understandings that arise through our relationships illuminate and shape the landscape of our experiences (Davies, 2011). We are born with the ability to express emotions such as anger, sadness, and joy, but it is through relationships that we learn how to accommodate these feelings to stress, loss, love, and other life events.

The capacity for intimacy and closeness is often impacted by stressful experiences. PTSD can leave individuals feeling disconnected from themselves and others, making it very difficult for them to cultivate closeness (Pitchford, 2009a). An individual who experiences a high degree of stress, and who struggles with relating to others may find her or himself overwhelmed with anxiety, avoiding connecting with others (Bartholomew & Horowitz, 1991). So, for individuals with PTSD, the anxiety they experience sets up a strong likelihood for detachment, leading to a lack of intimacy and a disconnection from others and even from themselves. As Paulson reflected, "We had to distance ourselves from any meaningful encounter with women because we felt that we could not share with them what we had experienced" (Paulson & Krippner, 2007, p. 66).

Let's also return to our college student, Sarah. After the rape, Sarah withdrew from others. Trust was stolen from her, and this loss impacted her ability to relate (or even want to relate) to others. She felt ashamed, alone, and without the strength necessary to overcome her traumatic encounter. The result was pulling back from others in the hope of finding some sense of safety and control.

### Intrapersonal and Interpersonal Isolation

From time to time, some form of isolation naturally occurs between individuals and others. However, there is an extremely deep level of isolation that can impact one's relationships to others and even to oneself. Intrapersonal isolation—the distancing of people from themselves—is a common reaction for individuals experiencing PTSD. The chaotic experiences of PTSD can leave individuals feeling cut off from themselves, feeling that they have lost their bearings and are adrift in a meaningless void. PTSD can also make them feel distant from others, even when surrounded by those who care about them. Such interpersonal isolation continues to prevail regardless of what, under other circumstances, could be positive encounters with others.

People with PTSD often experience a conflict between wishing to be separated from others while, at the same time, expressing a desire to connect with them (Herman, 1997). This ambivalence implies that the isolation incurred from trauma is both interpersonal and intrapersonal. This separation from themselves and others is increased when they re-experience the trauma through flashbacks—the images of the traumatizing event that suddenly intrude their daily thoughts (Pitchford, 2009a).

There are many approaches to understanding how isolation impacts people in connection to traumatic experiences. For example, the perception of death as a separation from oneself is an experience that is commonly experienced by those who are dying. But people who are consumed with the fear of dying commonly refer to their anxiety that the act of dying is a lonely experience. However, people who realize they are in a world that offers connections to themselves, to others, to a community, and even to pets may make two discoveries about death. First, they acknowledge that they are alone and helpless. Second, they can still derive meaning and joy from the relationships and experiences around them. This is highlighted in a Vietnam veteran's reflection upon his combat and homecoming experiences, and its affect upon his relationship to self and others, as recounted:

> He observed the death of "innocents" (e.g., women, children), became tormented by fear, sustained severe shrapnel wounds to the head, and held his

friend "in my arms as he bled to death" from an ambush. Vietnam was not the only "war" that the veteran had to encounter. On returning to the "States," he was welcomed with a reception of Americans spitting at him, disowning him, and accusing him of murder, and he had to endure his society's disorder of failing to support him and providing him with a shower of abandonment and hatred. He avoided relationships with women and became more and more consumed with drinking alcohol and isolating from others . . . Homeless and without a friend, he despaired. (Pitchford, 2009a, pp. 455–456)

This is also reflected in Teesha's case when she withdrew from others (an interpersonal reaction) and in how she lost interest in her own pursuits and life goals (an intrapersonal reaction).

### Guilt, Resentment, Abandonment, and Shame

It can be easy for someone with PTSD to resent those around her or him, to feel guilt at having survived the particular traumatizing event, or to experience abandonment not only by friends and family, but by one's country. Resentment may be experienced when someone with PTSD sees those without PTSD appearing "normal," while the traumatized individual remains in a world that does not seem to be safe or welcoming. Guilt may occur when the sole survivor of a motor vehicle accident reflects on how badly he misses his friends who met their untimely death. Abandonment often occurs when a rape victim is shunned because she is considered "damaged goods" by society. Shame can characterize a kidnapped person who had to perform daily sexual acts to survive captivity before she was released.

These feelings can often erupt in the form of anger or rage. For example, a combat veteran with PTSD may find herself returning stateside from a recent deployment, beginning to feel resentment at her family and or friends and how their lives appear to be untouched by the horrors of combat and war. She may wish that she could become unaware of the events that traumatized her, reconnecting to what her life was like prior to the trauma. She may lash out in verbal or physical aggression toward those around her, and they might have no idea why they have become targets of her rage.

Guilt can create a paradox for the trauma survivor. On the one hand, the survivor is fortunate that he or she escaped death, but on the other hand he or she would rather have died with his or her comrades. Survivor's guilt is especially intense when acts were committed that involved killing civilians, especially if they were women or children. Consider what Paulson's remembered as a survivor:

Plagued with guilt, I tried to find a place where I could go for forgiveness, to get away from this hell. I felt too guilty to go to God and church, for I had killed,

I had injured, and I had tortured my fellow human beings with intense delight. No, I could not go to God or church, for I had too much blood on my hands. I reasoned that no one wanted me now, not even God, for I had killed His children.

I felt completely alone and totally isolated. I lived in an alien world with which I could not communicate. I did not fit in with the other college students, since I was a Vietnam veteran, but I did not fit in with the military, either. I spent a little of my time studying, but most of my time I spent drinking to assuage the pain of life's all-too-obvious meaninglessness. The recurring visions and dreams of the killing I had seen and the killing I had done began to intensify. I just could not stop visualizing—and reliving—the emotional scenes of my comrades' deaths. Even the alcohol was not taking the edge off. I could not sleep, and I could not bear the pain of being awake. I could only suffer and hurt and despair over the meaninglessness and aloneness I endured, but even these were not as painful as the guilt. (Paulson & Krippner, 2007, p. 170)

Individuals with PTSD may also feel guilty if they believe that they had not endured enough traumas to warrant their strange behavior. Some combat veterans who only engaged in one battle were traumatized, but know of others who came through several battles with their psyches apparently unscathed. Needless to say, they have not heard of attachment theory or the predisposing stage of PTSD. These, and other, psychological dynamics explain the different reactions to combat. Also, it sometimes takes several years before PTSD symptoms manifest themselves; their combat buddies who appear in good spirits today might began to exhibit bizarre behaviors in a few years.

Another depressing experience is that of feeling abandoned. The sense of abandonment, rejection, and disregard can arrive when community members are distanced from the trauma survivor's stressful experiences. Veterans who served in Iraq or Afghanistan have reported returning to the states only to find that civilians are disillusioned about those conflicts, or worse, are indifferent and non-supportive, unaware of the realities being lived daily by U.S. men and women serving in foreign and hostile environments. The vulnerability of those leaving the battleground and returning home to such reactions can evoke both feelings of resentment and abandonment. Those veterans who are especially sensitive often feel rejected and misunderstood even though they stepped forward in bravery, fighting for what they were told was their country's cause.

Again, Daryl Paulson's reflections illuminate these elements through an encounter with his therapist:

When I first started to reveal to my therapist what I had done in Vietnam and how guilty I felt, I thought for sure that he, too, would abandon me. I could visually see him clutching his throat and gasping in horror as he fell from his chair over the disgusting, disgraceful things I had done in Vietnam. When I did tell him and felt he would kick me out of his office, he merely said, "Thank God that is out in the open now." He did not reject me. (Paulson & Krippner, 2007, p. 236)

Cambodian concentration camp survivors diagnosed with PTSD often expressed feelings of shame about their personal ordeals, especially if they had to collaborate with their captors to remain alive. It was common for them to experience a shame for their country as well as their identity as Cambodians. They knew that history would record the radical communists' genocide as one of the horrors of the 20th century, and they were ashamed to have been a part of it, even though they were not perpetrators.

### Alcohol and Substance Abuse

One of the most common "crutches" people with PTSD fall back upon is the frequent use/abuse of substances such as alcohol, prescription drugs, and illegal drugs. Many survivors of trauma use these mind-altering substances as a means to self-medicate from their oppressive symptoms of PTSD. The use of substances is often referred to we have termed a "co-morbid issue," the presence of two or more serious disorders such as both PTSD and substance abuse. There are a variety of substances people use to endure the agony of PTSD symptoms. They include, but are not limited to alcohol, marijuana, valium, klonopin, nicotine, heroin, cocaine, methamphetamine, with alcohol being the most common. A high percentage of people with PTSD have also been diagnosed or qualify for a diagnosis of alcohol abuse or, more seriously, dependence (Leeies, Pagura, Sareen, & Bolton, 2010). Paulson recalls his use of medication in moments of what existentialists refer to as complete *angst* or loss of meaning:

I tried to go on relaxing picnics with my friends, but I became too uneasy, even with the tranquilizers, to enjoy the picnic. I kept feeling that someone—the enemy—was hidden in the trees, stalking me, just as I had felt in Vietnam. At times, I became so tense and anxious on the picnics that I would have to drink a couple of belts of whiskey just to get through the ordeal. (Paulson & Krippner, 2007, p. 169)

Although it might provide immediate relief to anxiety, the use of alcohol as a means for coping can significantly impact a person's psychological and physical life, offering no long-lasting support toward the original provocation for use. If alcohol abuse is constant and occurs over a period of time, common impacts range from memory impairments, increased depression, decreased cognition, and the loss of pleasure, including sexual enjoyment, all of which could eventually result in a permanent impairment. Alcohol consumption can also increase the avoidance symptoms commonly found in PTSD (van der Kolk, 1987).

In the case of Michael, who we discussed earlier in this chapter, alcohol abuse led to dependence. As soon as he got out of bed in the morning, Michael needed a shot glass of whiskey to face the day. He always had a six-pack of beer on hand, and when a can or two of beer did not quell his anxiety, he returned to whiskey as well as rum, vodka, or whatever else was in his home bar. Teesha alleviated her symptoms through smoking marijuana, rationalizing her behavior by telling herself and others it was "medical weed," even though no physician was supervising its use. Before their traumatizing events, both Michael and Teesha enjoyed active sex lives. However, Teesha simply lost interest in sex and Michael was embarrassed when, in the company of the prostitutes he hired, he could not sexually perform.

In addition to the effects alcohol consumption can have upon PTSD, withdrawal from alcohol can increase the occurrence of trauma-related nightmares and hyperarousal. When a traumatized person attempts to cut back or stop substance use, the body needs time to accommodate its new chemical balance; in the meantime, the process of withdrawal can be excruciating and painful.

### Disturbed Sleep and Recurring Nightmares

Sleep is crucial in maintaining a healthy and balanced state of being. It provides excellent conditions for memory consolidation and transformation of disturbing memories over time (Payne & Kensinger, 2010). But an individual impacted by PTSD has a heightened level of stress that often impacts the ability to sleep through insomnia and other sleep disturbances as well as severe and persistent nightmares. It is also important to note the individual uniqueness of trauma survivors that is quite evident in disturbed sleep. As we consider how nightmares manifest in individuals diagnosed with PTSD, we will observe that there often was a previous history of sleep problems. Some men and women have lower resilience than others. Some people are extremely sensitive, having what psychologists often refer to as "thin boundaries," a correlate to nightmares even with those who do not have PTSD. And there are some individuals who suffer side effects from medication, one of the most frequent being the onset of frightening dreams (Pitchford, 2009b, p. 11).

Trauma survivors may experience two types of recurrent nightmares: traumatic (or trauma-related) and non-traumatic, the latter simply being "scary dreams." However, most people diagnosed with PTSD commonly experience traumatic nightmares (Pitchford, 2009b). Traumatic experiences create what is known as a "fear memory," which is a specific memory of the trauma combined with intense fear. This fear memory is extremely resistant to being integrated into the natural function of the brain and into the fabric of one's everyday life (Levin & Nielson, 2007; Pitchford, 2009b).

A non-traumatic nightmare is not evoked from a traumatic fear memory; rather, it is associated with negative and anxious experiences, such as the fear of giving a speech. This anxiety brings about major stimulation of the body during sleep. The defining point between the two types of nightmares is that non-traumatic nightmares are regulated through *extinction*—the systematic removal of emotional memories from the brain. Trauma-related nightmares, which cannot be processed through natural means of extinction, remain stuck (Pitchford, 2009b, p. 11). Thus, long-term sleep disturbances, such as nightmares, can produce significant distress for the trauma survivor. As one veteran stated:

> I am actually afraid to go to sleep at night. The nightmares are unbearable. My combat buddies died once in Iraq. But I have nightmares several times a week in which they are killed all over again. And I can still hear them screaming when I wake up. (Paulson & Krippner, 2007, p. 63)

### Loss of Identity and Meaning

A person's identity is built upon many influencing factors such as genetics, family of origin, sex and gender, social roles and cultural structures, personal myths, life scripts and worldviews, and internal working models. In addition, how individuals experience their day-to-day interactions with others and life circumstances can also affect their identity. "Who I am" and "What people think of me" are powerful voices, guiding this process. Through these influences, personal values and attitudes emerge, shaping the blueprint of one's identity. However, trauma can remove or destabilize what was once experienced as a solid ground, ripping out an individual's familiar sense of identity from his or her psyche. As Laura Brown (2008) noted:

> Trauma can shatter ... and evoke conflict by undermining previously held values, blocking the use of capacities emerging from a person's prior sense of self, and changing the face of the world as known, altering the parameters of the social context in which self is understood. (p. 51)

Let's revisit the case of Sarah. Her identity was built upon social contexts and cultural structures. She was a daughter, a college student, a girlfriend, and an ambitious learner with a promising future. Her own values were present as well: They included maintaining relationships, personal integrity, and fulfilling her commitments. When Sarah was raped, this changed everything. Trauma demolished her identity, leaving no familiar reference point that would enable her to reconstruct her identity. There was no internal working model, worldview, or personal myth available to help Sarah understand her traumatizing experience, or to derive meaning from it.

Attributing meaning to an event implies the creation of a rational or sensible structure. Cultural structures such as "Bad things sometimes happen to good people" and "Life is not a bowl of cherries" help some people become resilient following a dreadful life event. However, Sarah had never internalized such life scripts, clinging instead to a naïve personal mythology that "Everything works out for the best" and "This university is my haven of safety." The dissolution of a long-standing myth or structure causes many traumatized people to question the meaning of everything they do. The celebrated Russian novelist, Leo Tolstoy wrote books in which his characters frequently struggled with meaning. He termed this struggle a *life arrest*, and many people suffering from trauma would understand what Tolstoy meant by that term since their life has been "arrested" and stuck as a result of trauma.

Traumatizing events commonly challenge how survivors can derive meaning from the resulting traumatic experiences (Pitchford, 2009a). Deriving meaning from traumatic experiences is often challenged, as an air of senselessness surrounds those experiences. Making sense of senseless experiences is a massive challenge and can provoke incredible effort if one wants to live life more fully. The task is not an easy one. Making this attempt can be a very frightening step and considerable courage is required. As Herman (1997) accounted, traumatizing events "overwhelm the ordinary systems of care that give people a sense of control, connection, and meaning" (p. 33). Meaning then becomes a day-to-day struggle to survive the intrusive, the horrific, and the paralyzing world that has left survivors feeling there is no exit. Their lives have been arrested and there is no easy way to resume their journey.

Each of the four PTSD survivors presented in this chapter failed to derive positive meaning from their experiences even though some of them fought harder than others. Paulson sought to understand how to reconcile his combat experiences as well as his return to the states:

> Faced with the agony that there was no positive meaning (or Holy Grail) to be found in participation in Vietnam, I was thrown into an existential crisis. My entire world began to collapse. I could only suffer and drink and suffer and drink and suffer and drink. My world continued to fall apart, as I realized and felt to my core that my involvement in the war was for no positive purpose.

Over and over in my mind, I lamented how I had trusted the government and how it had betrayed me. Over and over, I asked myself, how could the politicians have done this to us? (Paulson & Krippner, 2007, p. 174)

Sarah struggled to regain her identity and to recover a sense of trust after the rape. Michael was left adrift in a sea of the haunting images of his wounded, dying, or dead patients. And Teesha continued to search for meaning in a world that she found was no longer safe.

There is no set path for making meaning; rather, it is an individual journey but one that can be embarked upon in the midst of support and guidance. Resources range from the support of family members and friends, to peers and therapeutic programs, to organized religion and personal faith. Oftentimes, such guidance needs to start from within, listening to the silent cries of the soul. But many trauma survivors struggle to breathe in their world of trauma, without a voice to call for help.

In conclusion, this chapter sketched quick portraits of four individuals whose worldviews were sundered by traumatizing events. Some people could have undergone similar incidents and come through them without flashbacks, nightmares, social isolation, extreme anxiety, or substance abuse. For them, the experiences would have been horrid, ghastly, and appalling but not traumatizing. But these individuals probably had life histories marked by strong attachments, flexible internal working models, adaptable personal myths, well-functioning coping styles, realistic worldviews, and—for all we know—genes that fostered resilience. Fortunately, there are interventions that can break the PTSD cycle, and these will be discussed in later chapters. Do not give up on Daryl, Sarah, Michael, and Teesha; we will discover where they went as they continued their life passages.

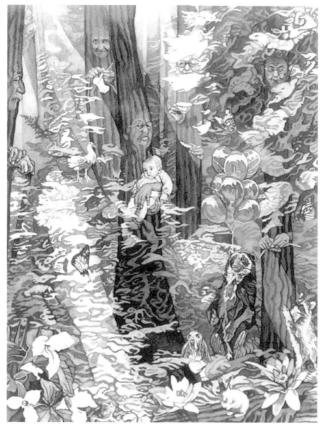

Grandma Trees (Reproduced from the original art of Dierdre Luzwick.)

# 6

# The Neuroscience of PTSD

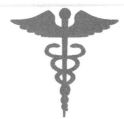

Now that we have begun to understand how post-traumatic stress disorder influences individual attitudes and behaviors, it is time to "pull back the veil" and peer into the chemical and biological relationships that accompany PTSD symptoms. PTSD interacts with a network of brain systems (such as the amygdala and hippocampus) that communicate through messages given in chemical signals. These messenger cells, called neurotransmitters, permit the emergence of a potent process of understanding as it is framed and orchestrated through an individual's experience of the trauma. And, as noted previously, these experiences often are built upon a person's past experiences, either positive or negative, that serve as predisposing factors for PTSD.

There might even be genetic predispositions to PTSD. One study of Holocaust survivors' children noted that, like their parents, they displayed unusually low levels of the hormone cortisol, a deficit of which often is associated with PTSD (Yehuda and Bierer, 2007). This study claimed to have eliminated child-parent relationships as the reason for this hormonal imbalance. In another study, Swedish soldiers serving in Bosnia and Herzegovina with low pre-service salivary cortisol levels had a higher risk of developing PTSD than those with normal pre-service cortisol levels (Lindley, et al., 2004). In both instances, cortisol is important in restoring homeostasis, or balance, following a stressful event. However, there is no one-to-one relationship between cortisol levels and PTSD;

this is only one aspect of a larger structure, one in which the nervous system plays a primary role.

The nervous system is a network of specialized cells called neurons; a second set of cells—the glial cells—provide nutrition, insulation, and support for the neurons. As their name implies, glial cells seem to "glue" the neurons together. The nervous system coordinates the activities of humans and other animals, and transmits signals between different parts of the body. There are two major branches of the nervous system. One of them is the central nervous system (CNS) consisting of the brain, spinal cord, and (surprisingly) the retina of the eye. The second branch of the CNS is the peripheral nervous system (PNS) consisting of sensory neurons, neuron clusters called ganglia, and additional neurons connecting them to each other and to the CNS.

Sensory neurons are vital to such senses as taste, smell, sight, hearing, touch, balance, pain, kinesthesia, and several others. (There are many more senses than the traditional "five senses" still cited in many elementary schools.) Neurons send signals by means of the previously mentioned neurotransmitters. When a cell receives a signal it may become excited, inhibited, or changed in some other way. Serotonin is an example of a neurotransmitter that excites the nervous system, while encephalin is an example of a neurotransmitter that inhibits the nervous system. Encephalin is the body's natural "opiate" and people who become opium or heroin addicts lose the capacity of this natural way (simply stated, the natural capacity) to calm the mind and body.

By the way, the so-called "mind" and "body" work so closely together that we often use the term "mind-body" to demonstrate this collaboration. And we often use the word "psyche" to describe mind-body functions that have very deep meanings associated with them, "psyche" being the Greek word for "soul."

Many behaviors associated with PTSD can be traced to the activity of neurotransmitters. For example, an unpleasant memory can activate the amygdala's "fight or flight" response, inducing the release of the neurotransmitter norepinephrine from the adrenal glands, hyperarousing the entire mind-body system. This "overactive adrenaline response" can create brain patterns that persist long after the event that triggered the original response, making an individual hyperresponsive to similar situations in the future.

The peripheral nervous system can be further subdivided into the sympathetic nervous system (SNS), which triggers the "fight or flight" response and can suffer from wear and tear if this response is overused. The parasympathetic nervous system (PSNS) performs housekeeping functions for the entire nervous system as well as conserving energy so that the organism will be able to function smoothly and efficiently. The field of neuroscience studies the nervous system and all of its subdivisions, many—but not all—of which we have described here.

(For example, the PSNS has two branches, the sensory and the motor, and the motor branch subdivides into the autonomic and the somatic nervous systems.) Just take our word for it; the nervous system, especially in humans, is a many-splendored thing!

We should add that there are many more bodily systems. The immune system's cells, tissues, and organs protect the body against microorganisms that might cause infectious disease. The endocrine system consists of glands that secrete hormones; these hormones do not act as quickly as neurotransmitters but their effects are usually longer-lasting. Knowledge of this relationship is especially important for therapists working with PTSD patients whose ability to function sexually has been impaired due to interactions among the psyche, the nervous system, the endocrine system, and the immune system.

## STRESS AND STRESSORS

The word "stress" has been borrowed by psychology and medicine from physics and engineering. It describes the attempts, both successful and unsuccessful, of an organism to respond adequately to emotional and physical demands, real or imagined. What is known as the "generalized stress response" first begins with an alarm that might trigger a "fight or flight" response; secondly, the organism resists the stress, but if this fails, the third step is exhaustion. Events that produce stress responses are called "stressors," and people in all cultures have had to cope with them.

Typically, these stressors do not traumatize people who have developed healthy ways of coping with stress. The stressor is usually a taxing event that is integrated into the course of one's life. For others, however, the event has a traumatizing effect on a person and becomes a traumatic experience. Some people rebound quickly from a stressor such as a motor vehicle accident, left with nothing but a disturbing memory of that event. For others, that same event becomes traumatizing, resulting in a traumatic experience that could lead to PTSD or a related stress disorder.

Remember that stress responses can be evoked by either real or imagined stimuli; this is why it is important to separate events from experiences. Events are objective; everyone involved will describe them in more or less the same way. Experiences are subjective and allow for the imagination to create demons and goblins, fears and horrors, and suspicions and attributions that may have no existence outside of one's personal fantasies and beliefs. For example, throughout history, entire societies have conjured stress-related responses to imaginary stimuli. This has led to inquisitions, witch hunts, and holocausts, that were based more on fantasy than fact.

Understanding the human brain is a challenge because of its complexity. It is a living organ that, over the course of evolution, adapted to changes in climate, food supplies, and natural catastrophes. This capacity for change is known as *neuroplasticity*. The brain has its own set of natural, biological rules that maintain a harmony necessary for the maintenance of a bodily system, either human or non-human. However, if any one of these rules is broken, the repercussions can be profound.

PTSD is one of these rule-breakers imposing its own agenda upon the body's natural neurological system, literally overwhelming the brain's system of communication through altering its chemical pathways and processes. The biology of ordinary, routine stress responses and the biology of trauma are fundamentally different. Stress unleashes a cascade of biological and neurological changes, but the body returns to its normal ways of functioning after the stressor is gone. For most types of stress, the organism's natural balance will be re-established once the stress has been successfully managed. In contrast, the effects of PTSD exist long after the stressor has disappeared.

A major problem accompanying PTSD is the individual's fixation on the traumatizing event (or events). When individuals experience what seems to be a life-threatening incident, they immediately go into what is termed a "survival and self-protection" mode. Most people quickly regain their equilibrium, but those who develop PTSD do not return to a natural state. They remain vigilant, constructing exaggerated habits of self-protection and becoming hyperaware of their surroundings, always on the lookout for something that will remind them of the threat. As a result, it is important to understand the processes that keep individuals from returning to a state of comfort, and remain haunted by their trauma.

There are many reasons for this inability to bounce back, but what they have in common is that the usual means of coping do not alleviate the stress. Most people rely on their psychological and physical resiliency, support from friends with whom they can discuss the stressor, gym workouts or other forms of exercise, meditation or prayer, and various additional methods and practices. You may be happy to know that sexual activity can be a potent stress reliever. Even if these activities are available to the PTSD sufferer, they do not alleviate the stress because they are ineptly applied or attempted too late.

## THE VIRUS IN THE COMPUTER SYSTEM

A person's ability to cope with stress depends upon the maturity and flexibility of the individual's nervous system, his or her personality structure, and one's previous reactions to stressors. The way people respond to stressors determines whether these stressors remain unpleasant events or whether they have the capacity to traumatize the person experiencing them. The same event will become a traumatic experience for some people, but merely a disturbing memory for others, one that they assimilate into their life story. Some people even find humor in the stressor: being trapped in an elevator for hours can be reframed as an experiment in sensory isolation, losing one's savings to a fraudulent investor can be retold as their contribution to the "culture of sleaze," and being sexually harassed at work for several months can become a scenario for an imaginary stage play with well-known actors cast as the villains.

An individual's personal myths and belief systems can prevent or foster the development of PTSD. Being able to manage stress by falling back on one's resources is often called relying on an "internal locus of control." Using problem-focused coping strategies helps to reduce the possibility of PTSD developing; this ability is often referred to as "being mindful." Both mindfulness and self-regulation serve as "buffers" that help people to manage stress.

Let's imagine a computer system that represents the human body and mind. This system maintains an effective level of performance through the support of a central processor, namely the brain. This processor serves as the regulator of such basic functions as eating, sleeping, and walking. If a virus were to threaten any single part of the central processor, then the entire system would be impacted. This virus would, by its nature, infect the system, compromising its ability to thrive or even to survive. The central processor would then automatically put the secure parts of the system into a "safe mode" that ensures survival. Even so, performance is dramatically diminished and sometimes the system can never fully recover. Substitute the word "trauma" for the word "virus" and you can fathom the catastrophic effects that can put the "central processor," or brain, at risk.

When people endure a series of traumatizing experiences and develop PTSD, this disorder represents their best possible effort to recover. When a computer is badly damaged by viruses, a new one can be purchased to take its place. But human beings cannot make a substitution this easily; they need to find other means of recovery or live the rest of their lives in a restricted, diminished state of functioning. However, seeing PTSD as a normal and natural response to what we would consider an abnormal and unnatural situation lays the groundwork for the human psyche's reconstruction through psychotherapy and counseling. It also downplays such words as "disorder" and "mental illness" that are applied to a condition that reminds us of the fragility of the human species.

## WHAT HAPPENS TO THE BRAIN DURING PTSD?

A person's biological response to a trauma, and, in many cases, the subsequent development of PTSD, depends greatly upon the way that he or she interprets the potentially traumatizing event. And this interpretation is heavily influenced by the way that the person reacted to stressors in the past. These earlier reactions are especially evident when a negative response to trauma renders an individual helpless, terrified, and fearful. All of these reactions involve the brain and body's neurological and chemical reactions. Indeed, PTSD has deleterious effects on the body's central and peripheral nervous systems, as well as their various branches.

Ordinarily, a person's brain develops with reliance upon a balance of communication from the neurotransmitters, or messenger neurons that exist throughout the body—not only in the brain, but also in the heart and gut. Gradually, a natural brain function achieves harmony between the brain and the body. The natural defenses of the brain regulate stress, especially during emergencies, illnesses, and life transitions. However, there are extraordinary life encounters that can evoke a breakdown in a person's healthy functioning.

Individuals with PTSD display changes in the way in which the brain communicates with the body. The body and brain try to integrate the stressful events with past experiences. What was seen, heard, smelled, touched, and felt is cast into a pre-existing mode; if no such mold is easily available, the brain keeps trying to find a suitable match. And if no such match exists, the event becomes traumatic and the individual keeps reliving it, attempting in vain to integrate it into his or her personal narrative. This reliving is triggered by the parasympathetic nervous system (PSNS), the bodily system that regulates such processes as stimulation.

Most people have a rest period after experiencing PSNS-evoked arousal but for people with PTSD, these rest periods are few and far between. In PTSD, the system is overwhelmed, over-stimulating the brain, especially the bean-shaped amygdala, which responds to such neurotransmitters as norepinephrine and epinephrine. At the same time, vivid memories are aroused in the seahorse-shaped hippocampus and remind people with PTSD of their trauma. There is no easy escape; alcoholism and substance abuse are examples of medicating oneself that may provide temporary relief, but no long-term solution.

Let's take a closer look at these important parts of the brain. A key function of the amygdala is the regulation of emotional responses such as fear. The amygdala is not stimulated by recall or imagery alone, but can also be activated by visual perception. As a result, facial expressions and environmental cues may trigger flashbacks; a lecherous grin may remind someone who has been raped of his or her assailant; an exploding firecracker may result in a combat veteran ducking for cover in any available gulley or ditch. Hence, in the case of PTSD, amygdala activity is overly reactive to any stimulus that is remotely connected to the traumatic experience (Pitchford, 2009, p. 123).

As for the hippocampus, it plays an essential role not only in encoding and processing memories, but in the retention of unique and overwhelming experiences (Levin & Nielson, 2007). It plays a major role in locating a memory of an event in time, place, and context. As a result, when people with PTSD find themselves in a similar locale to the one producing the traumatizing event, an unbearable emotional reaction may occur. Further, the hippocampus is a fairly small organ; it is constantly packaging and transmitting memories to areas in the cerebral cortex where more space is available. A well-functioning hippocampus "clears the deck" each day to process new experiences, each with its own emotional component.

To be anatomically correct, we should refer to both the amygdala and the hippocampus in the plural as each hemisphere in the brain contains one. The amygdalae (to use the plural form) are collections of nuclei, not individual organs. They help to activate the sympathetic nervous system (SNS) and assist in the manufacture of such brain chemicals as norepinephrine, epinephrine, and dopamine. The hippocampae (to use the plural form) are the parts of the brain most vulnerable to stress, and can even atrophy, or "dry up," when excessively stimulated. They play a key role in consolidating short-term memories into long-term memories, which accounts for the wear and tear that they suffer when dealing with traumatizing events. The amygdala (reverting to the more familiar singular form) also plays a key role in memory consolidation. A dramatic event is integrated into the memory bank gradually, not immediately. If the hippocampus, amygdala, and other parts of the brain cannot successfully consolidate the horror, these events end up becoming traumatic experiences.

The signals to the PSNS can be subtle or overt. For example, if someone was physically assaulted during a summer evening, something as subtle as a cricket chirp could produce an anxiety response and that person could become hyperaroused. Hyperarousal is a constant state of being "on guard" against being harmed again by another traumatizing event. As a result, that person's arousal processes become overwhelmed. Again, this is a normal, natural response to an abnormal, unnatural situation. The mind-brain does its best to cope with stress, but its best is not good enough to stall the onset of PTSD.

People with PTSD have trouble navigating the emotions that are provoked in reaction to their experiences, and manifest difficulties learning how to find a renewed state of balance. A functional person becomes hyperaroused when a threat to his or her person is detected. At the time of the threat, the person then decides to encounter it (fight) or run from it (flight). As we have said before, this is known as the "fight or flight" response. However, in some instances including PTSD, a person may simply freeze, being unable to make a decision whether to fight or to flee.

Common hyperarousal responses include quick startle responses such as becoming angry, anxious, or fearful, as well as sleep disturbances, evoked because hyperaroused people have trouble falling asleep. Such responses are instigated through various mechanisms within the limbic system of the brain, namely the amygdala, hippocampus, and neighboring parts of the cerebral cortex referred to as the "prefrontal cortex." These areas do not work together as a perfectly synchronized system; instead, each of them attempts, in its own way, to regulate emotion, arousal, memory, and several other related functions. At the same time, the continued stimulation of the brain's fear and memory regions (basically, the amygdala and hippocampus) evoke the all too common hyperarousal reactions seen in individuals diagnosed with PTSD.

When trauma is captured in memory before it is completely processed, and when one gets stuck in those memories, the hippocampus provides the common, instant replay of many elements of the traumatizing event. This is referred to as the "re-experiencing" phenomenon often associated with PTSD. Re-experiencing can take the form of partial recollections from triggers such as the smells, sounds, and body sensations associated with the experience, sometimes leading to a full-fledged flashback—an unexpected revisitation of particular moments from the traumatic experience or experiences.

A traumatized couple who has lost their infant baby to an infectious disease may experience a flashback to that child when hearing children happily playing in a nearby park. A combat veteran who comes home after witnessing the killing of children may respond with inappropriate fear and anxiety upon hearing the sounds of children at play in that same park because those sounds are reminiscent of those heard when children were dying.

The flashback experience was vividly portrayed in the film, *The Last Samurai*, when Tom Cruise's character, Nathan Algren, is a passenger on a ship to Japan. He stands in front of the mirror, looking at himself, preparing to don his military uniform. Just as he completes making the finishing touches on his ensemble, he flashes back to the moments of combat that have always haunted him. He returns the uniform to its case and begins to drown his memories in glass after glass of whiskey.

Another example can be seen in the behavior of Brad Pitt's character, Tristan Ludlow, in the film, *Legends of the Fall*. After failing to save his brother, Samuel, from being killed in combat, Tristan returns home to find himself haunted by his memories. Samuel had been rendered helpless by mustard gas and stumbled into barbed wire. Tangled in the wire, German soldiers took advantage of the situation and shot Samuel; Tristan made a rescue attempt but was too late. We find Tristan rendered completely numb, traumatized, and wandering from war zone to war zone. He returns home, changed—and not for the better. On one particular day, he finds a calf caught in the barbed wire perimeter of the farm. Upon trying to save the calf, Tristan's invisible wounds come alive, and he instantly finds himself holding his dying brother in his arms.

Sometimes a traumatizing event seems to have been assimilated because one's symptoms have lessened. Later, however, the individual discovers that the condition has not really disappeared. Even decades later, the body's responses may remain the same as if the threat were just around the corner. This is especially characteristic of hyperaroused states, which are often accompanied by the re-experiencing of the trauma. Prompts and cues while one is awake may lead to flashbacks, or to recurring nightmares that replay the traumatic experience. Also, PTSD has been found to alter neurotransmitter levels, and this leaves traumatized individuals with heightened levels of stress accompanied by increased cortisol levels. It may also lead to severe depression associated with a deficit of the mood-altering neurotransmitter serotonin.

There may be other specific biochemical changes that influence traumatized individuals' responses to their environment, changes that may trigger a chemical reaction. As a result, the brain becomes more susceptible to fear, anxiety, anger, or depression. Such neurotransmitters as serotonin and such hormones as cortisol, as well as other brain chemicals, are stimulated beyond what would be expected, thereby re-enforcing, as it were, the recall and response that PTSD invokes. Such responses, if repeated, create a greater possibility for an individual with PTSD to develop health problems due to weakened immune functioning.

A small amount of stress may enhance a worker's productivity, an athlete's performance, or a writer's creativity. Indeed, Hans Selye (1974) used the terms "eustress" and "distress" to discriminate between helpful and harmful stress. But post-traumatic stress (or distress) has no redeeming virtues and plenty of drastic consequences.

## THE NEUROSCIENCE OF NIGHTMARES

Sleep is important for the maintenance of bodily balance or homeostasis. If individuals are deprived of adequate sleep, their day-by-day functioning will be diminished. A nightmare is an experience that provokes terror in people to the point of suddenly awakening them (Hartmann, 1984; Levin & Nielson, 2007). But a nightmare may also occur at sleep onset, thereby affecting and delaying the initiation of sleep. Nightmares usually incorporate horrifying and discomforting details into their scenarios.

As we mentioned earlier, the difference between typical, non-traumatic nightmares and those that become recurrent trauma-related nightmares is that the latter disrupt the sleep cycle and can cause long-term sleep disorders such as insomnia or narcolepsy. Dopamine, which sometimes acts as a neurotransmitter and sometimes as a hormone (a brain chemical with a longer-lasting effect than a neurotransmitter), can influence the onset of nightmares or even support nightmare activity in general.

The sleep cycle, ranging from light to deep sleep, may be severely impacted by sleep disturbances for individuals with PTSD. These individuals can be effortlessly aroused from sleep by nightmares that re-enact the traumatic experiences, usually in great detail. In fact, the neurochemistry of nightmares is connected not only with disrupted sleep, but with interrupted daytime behavior (for example, hyperarousal) as well.

One explanation for this connection is found in the neurotransmitter serotonin, which seems to play multiple roles in the central nervous system including the regulation of sleep. Serotonin plays a role in other psychophysiological changes as well, including the regulation of aggression, the maintenance of a healthy appetite, well-functioning cardiovascular and respiratory activity, and changes in mood.

As we have stated before, it is important to remember when considering the formation of nightmares in people diagnosed with PTSD that every individual is unique in his or her capacity to cope with traumatic experiences. In addition, you will recall that PTSD is a series of steps on a continuum of stress disorders, and people on the low end of the continuum have fewer and less disturbing nightmares than those on the far end. If the person's mind-body system is characterized by low resilience, exceptionally thin psychological boundaries, or adverse medication side effects, these factors can contribute to the onset of nightmares (Pitchford, 2009, p. 123). Predisposing factors such as emotional deprivation in childhood, being bullied in high school, or having a history of work harassment can also increase the frequency of trauma-related nightmares.

Memories of trauma can become ingrained and evoke repetitive nightmares that are very difficult to modify. In the case of most nightmares, no major trauma has been experienced, but perhaps another type of horrible experience may have transpired, such as rejection by a romantic partner. That experience may have evoked anxiety and became linked to major stimulation during sleep.

Trauma-related nightmares are associated with numerous conflicts in areas of the brain that contribute to emotional processes such as the regulation of emotional responses (Pitchford, 2009). The control and occurrence of trauma-related nightmares is regulated by the amygdala and the hippocampus. Alterations in these two limbic regions involve amplified activity through steady stimulation. Nightmares take form when arousal and distress are continually stimulated (and exaggerated) in the amygdala; this is often paired with related traumatic memories within the hippocampus. The brain incessantly makes attempts to resolve or diminish this stimulation; however, it is unsuccessful due to continual triggering of the memories. It is during sleep that this exaggeration combines its efforts with memories associated with the trauma and elicits what is known as a traumatic nightmare experience (Pitchford, 2009, p. 123).

During "normal" dreaming experiences, amygdala activity differs, based upon the expressed level of emotion; however, the stimulus level for fear responses is surprisingly low. A small amount of stimulation of the amygdala during dreaming may generate anxiety, though, with trauma-related nightmares, amygdala activity is continually stimulated, resulting in extreme states of fearfulness and anxiety.

Most nightmares occur in the sleep stage known as REM, or rapid eye movement sleep. Dreams can also occur without the presence of REM, but REM dreams tend to be more vivid and emotional. There are more reports of unpleasant dreams than pleasant dreams, indicating that the mind-body system is functioning well, processing emotion, and purging or altering the negative moods that occurred during the day.

Sleep does more than consolidate memories. It also transforms them in ways that might be less accurate but more useful and adaptive, even fostering new insights (Payne & Kensinger, 2010, p. 293). In dreaming, the hippocampus relays some aspects of memory through novel, unexpected, and sometimes bizarre situations based upon word meanings (especially metaphors), symbols (usually expressed as visual images), and memory fragments. However, when nightmares rooted in traumatizing events are experienced, the dreaming process usually portrays these events realistically, in a manner that is quite close in accuracy to the original traumatizing event or the resulting traumatic experience (Barrett & Behbehani, 2003).

## FEAR MEMORIES AND DREAMS

The hippocampus plays a crucial role in regulating emotions in dreams and nightmares and in facilitating the extinction of fear. The hippocampus and amygdala control several ways fear memories are expressed. People who have recurrent dreams usually report content that is commonly connected with emotional processes. In individuals diagnosed with PTSD, their nightmare experiences are immersed in extreme amygdala stimulation connected with persistent flooding of memories of the traumatizing events. Also, amygdala activity is amplified during nightmare experiences, which overwhelms its function by increasing fear responses. Fear conditioning and the process of managing fear arousal within nightmare experiences involve multiple components working together, such as *fear memories*, which combine amygdala stimulation with image retrieval from the hippocampus (Pitchford, 2009, p. 124).

Fear memories are a common occurrence in both ordinary dreams and terrifying nightmares. They occur within the realm of memory functioning, typically becoming pathological or intrusive, as in nightmares, only when they occur on such a consistent basis as to overwhelm the limbic system. Naturally, the limbic system and other areas of the brain handle such experiences effectively, processing emotions and their corresponding memories to allow for the preparation, by means of dreaming, of the next day's round of experiences.

Fear memories, however, become more intrusive when they resist extinction. That is, individuals with PTSD are considered more vulnerable to having nightmares due to their intensely charged and vivid fear memories around their traumatic experiences. This vulnerability interrelates with sleep's neurophysiology and then continually stimulates the already charged fear memories, creating greater resistance to eradication (Levin & Nielson, 2007).

In the case of ordinary dreaming, fear memories may become triggered, but they are quickly integrated through extinction; this process inhibits their ability to transform into nightmares and fortifies the body's natural ability to prevent future fear memories from developing. However, the dreaming process is not linear or simplistic. Since dreams vary in their context, their content, and their unique subjectivity, the limbic system is always working to manage and modulate the continuous stream of fear memories and other processes initiated in the course of dreaming.

Let's return to our discussion of the film character, Nathan Algren, in *The Last Samurai*. Another scene from the film depicts this character being haunted by his combat experiences through nightmares. We see this when Algren often wakes up demanding *sake*, a potent alcoholic beverage common in Japan, to help extinguish his painful memories. This occurs both during his time as a prisoner of war and while he is trying to detoxify himself from alcohol. As noted, biological and chemical changes often occur in individuals who experience trauma, so it is no surprise that sleep patterns are erratic and that nightmares occur frequently. Some of the possible contributors to Nathan's sleep problems are his nightmares and his continued thoughts around his traumatic experiences, such as his feelings of guilt for killing children.

In the film, Nathan's nightmares are intense enough that he often awakens from his sleep, which suggests a couple of possible issues. One is that the shame, guilt, and anxiety Nathan has infused into his traumatic experiences are no doubt exhibited in his nightmares. However, these awakenings can affect the quality of sleep, eventually depriving the body of the neurochemical processing and rest that is needed to maintain full awareness the following day. In addition, Nathan's overall physical health deteriorates as well as his psychological functioning.

## PTSD AND MEMORY

PTSD impacts memory in wakefulness as well as in sleeping and dreaming. PTSD memories differ from ordinary waking memories in many ways. We have already discussed fear memories and how they are easily triggered by environmental cues. It is difficult for someone to describe these memories in words because they are filled with imagery, emotion, and bodily sensations. Therefore, it is probably easier for someone to dream about a traumatic experience than to describe it when awake. Furthermore, these memories are often fragmented and cannot be described in a linear narrative in the way that most experiences can be discussed as if they were a story (Vasterling & Brewin, 2005).

PTSD, especially in childhood, can have lasting effects on the hippocampus, which is especially vulnerable to fear memories and can be damaged by recurring trauma, whether it be rape or combat. The brain's medial prefrontal cortex plays a key role in memory, sending signals to the amygdala, whose cluster of nerve cells store memories. But people with PTSD demonstrate a decrease in the prefrontal cortex's blood flow, and this probably interferes with its communication with the amygdala (Sapolsky, 1996). Ordinarily, the prefrontal context calms the fears, but if the blood supply is impaired, this function is blocked. Hence, fear memories do not get properly integrated either in wakefulness or in sleep. They are like undigested food that clogs up the stomach, evoking feelings of pain and discomfort. The result of this "indigestion" is chronic fear, panic attacks, anxiety, and phobias. These phobias can range from fear of open spaces to fear of closed spaces, from fear of noises to fear of silence.

The disruption of memory and other information processing in the brain is central to understanding PTSD. One's traumatic experiences and their aftermath are rooted in the interplay among the amygdala, the hippocampus, and the prefrontal cortex. In most people, this dance proceeds smoothly and harmoniously, but in PTSD the dance becomes chaotic, the harmony becomes noisy static, and the beauty of a well-functioning brain becomes a horror story from the scariest film scenario. And the horror never stops; it takes different forms at night than it does during the day, but people with severe PTSD cannot escape its grasp.

Children with PTSD have trouble learning, adults with PTSD have difficulty in holding a job or maintaining a relationship, and people of all ages often *dissociate*. They try to escape the traumatic experiences by forgetting segments of them, or by retreating into fantasy (Bremner & Marmar, 1998). When people dissociate, they break the ordinary flow of thought, memory, and behavior. They separate some mental processes from others, for example, crying while telling a funny story, or laughing while viewing a sad movie. Extreme forms of dissociation include feeling that one has left one's body, that one is in a different time or place, or that one is actually a different person. Because people with PTSD are not able to live in the "here and the now," their short-term memory is often impaired. They might learn a new skill one day, and completely forget what they have learned the following day. Children with PTSD sometimes have trouble learning how to ride a bicycle, how to play a videogame, or how to play a musical instrument. What is learned one day is forgotten a few hours later. This is often called *dissociative amnesia*, a loss of memory due to temporary or frequent dissociation.

People with PTSD often demonstrate problems with *declarative memory*. They cannot recall lists of basic facts such as the months of the year, or the order of cards while playing a game. They do very poorly when putting something in order and following a sequence is important. But other types of memory are affected as well, such as motor memory (as when driving an automobile), and long-term memory (which may make it difficult for them to accurately recall a traumatizing event). Sometimes a person will "suddenly remember" being raped by a family member decades ago, but it is hard to determine if these memories are fantasies, symbolic representations of some other type of abuse, or the recall of actual events. Memory is not a videotape in the brain that accurately records every lived event; memory is more like a merry-go-round that picks up and drops off passengers as it makes its perpetual circle.

## LEAH'S STORY

There are numerous examples from everyday life of people with PTSD who display the behaviors we have described in this chapter. Leah was born on the island of Mindanao in the Philippines, the site of Muslim separatist activity. For decades, the Muslim Abu Saydf militants have tortured, kidnapped, and killed villagers as well as the government soldiers sent to crush the insurrection. Leah's family left Mindanao as soon as her father could find employment in the provinces on another island, but not before Leah had been raised in a culture of fear. One never knew when one's house would be broken into by marauding militants or when a neighbor with a little money would be seized and held for ransom. We would consider these as predisposing factors in what later turned out to be a case of PTSD.

Leah enjoyed her new home, but still had occasional nightmares concerning masked gunmen who invaded her house, even though this never had occurred in waking life. Leah obtained good grades in school, and the occasional nightmares seemed to be the only residue of her earlier experience. However, her parents were concerned because she did not have much of an appetite. Also, Leah was suspicious of strangers and was reluctant to socialize with her classmates. Her parents attributed this behavior to adolescent modesty and did not make a connection between these behaviors and her childhood years in Mindanao.

When Leah was a student in high school, she had several altercations with a teacher, Miss Concepcion. Leah was quite bright, especially in the field of history, which was one of courses taught by Miss Concepcion. Leah made the mistake of correcting Miss Concepcion when the teacher referred to the Filipino patriot José Rizal as Joseph Rizal. The two names are equivalent but Rizal never went by the name of Joseph. Leah did not correct her teacher in front of the class, but only in private, thinking that she was being helpful. She also corrected her teacher's confusion of several historic names such as former Presidents Macapagal and Magsayay, and also corrected Miss Concepcion's mispronunciation of names of non-Filipinos who had played an important role in the country's history, Magellan and MacArthur, among them.

Two months into the term, Miss Concepcion struck back. She started to punish Leah for any minor infraction of rules, such as making Leah stand in the hallway for whispering in class, or repeatedly writing on a full sheet of paper "I will not be late for school." She began to refer to Leah as "Miss Know-It-All" and made derogatory remarks about Leah's habitual shyness. For example, Miss Concepcion would taunt Leah by such comments as "You won't find a man if you pretend to know more than he does." "What real man would want to choose a simple wallflower like you?" For better or for worse, Leah did not share these incidents of abuse with her parents, knowing that they were simple folk from the country and would merely assume that the teacher knew best.

Each of these insults became a fear memory for Leah, and she felt her heart pound and her breaths quicken whenever Miss Concepcion was nearby. Physical punishment was allowed at Leah's school, if the occasion demanded it. Miss Conception beat Leah with a small stick trying to rid her of the "pride" that was the teacher's term for Leah's intelligence. But sometimes Leah felt that these beatings on her hands would be preferable to the contempt she encountered whenever her gaze met that of her antagonistic teacher.

For a class assignment, Leah wrote a term paper about a Filipino president she had greatly admired, Corazon "Cory" Aquino. She received a low grade on the essay, even though her classmates thought it was a fine piece of work. When Leah asked Miss Concepcion what was wrong with the paper, she was told, "There is too much exaggeration in this paper. You wrote about Cory as if she were a saint. Only the church has the right to decide who deserves sainthood. Besides, your point of view distracts girls from their future roles as obedient wives and devoted mothers. This is the proper role model for Filipinas to follow."

This frontal attack on Leah's attempt to write an essay about her heroine might be seen as the instigator of what was to come—the activating factor in her PTSD. Leah began to have nightmares several times a week; her attackers were no longer masked men, but unmasked female teachers, all of whom bore a resemblance to Miss Concepcion. In the Philippines, teachers usually focus their disciplinary measures against boys who are less docile in the classroom, so Miss Concepcion's behavior seemed out of place. In some of the nightmares, Miss Concepcion was demeaning Leah while the boys in the classroom were running rampant. While awake, this bizarre state of affairs violated Leah's personal myth that teachers were fair and impartial, and that she was living in a just world where hard work and honesty would yield both individual and professional rewards. The violation of these personal myths had a devastating effect upon Leah. She trembled whenever entering the history classroom. Leah stopped participating in class discussions as she felt that she could not fight back or flee the antagonism she faced.

Leah's health had always been good, but now she began to have bouts of high fevers and influenza. In PTSD, the breakdown of the immune system may precede other deleterious effects as it did with Leah. Later, she withdrew from her few friends in school and her grades began to decline. But what seemed to be lethargy was actually a hyperaroused state; Leah began to become suspicious of her friends and abruptly dropped them. She began to complain about the low level of instruction in her school and that it really was not worth the trouble to apply herself to her homework.

For the first time in her life, Leah began to drink alcohol to excess, starting with the local Ginebra San Miguel beer and ultimately proceeding to a popular brandy, Grand Matador. Leah's parents berated her but she shunned their advice, telling them they were as bad as Miss Concepcion. What she did not tell them was that she had been hearing Miss Concepcion's voice scolding her even when she was not in school. Imbibing alcohol was Leah's attempt to drown out the harsh rebukes, as well as the occasional flashbacks to her constant putdowns in the history classroom. Here we have several examples of factors that used the PTSD symptoms: withdrawal, low performance, and substance abuse.

Finally, Leah's behavior became apparent to the school officials and she was referred to counseling. Leah admitted to the counselor that her attitude had changed drastically and that she was praying for an "inspiration" that would put her back on track. Her counselor did not deny the importance of inspiration, but began to explore the conflict between Leah's belief system, the violation of those beliefs, and her resulting destructive behavior. Her counselor spent considerable time focusing on Leah's substance abuse. If she continued on the path to alcoholism, it would be deleterious to her immune system, hormonal system, nervous system, as well as to her psyche. And this attempt to save her soul provided the most important motivation for Leah's ultimate rehabilitation. It also was fortunate that Leah was transferred out of Miss Concepcion's class.

Not all children are as fortunate. The effects of trauma on childhood memories have important implications. Children who live in war zones or in crime-ridden cities witness violence frequently, and may even be victims themselves. Their academic performance is likely to suffer because of the negative effect that trauma has on both short-term and long-term memories. This chapter has illuminated the close connection between mental and physiological aspects of PTSD, and why both aspects of what we have called the mind-body need to be considered when attempting to rehabilitate an individual with a diagnosis of PTSD.

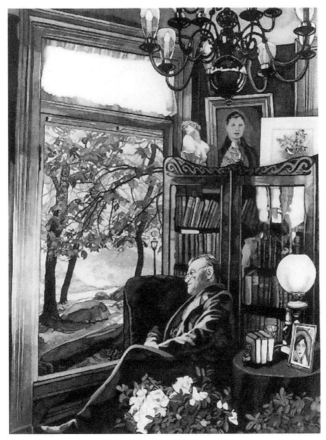

Jennie Kissed Me (Reproduced from the original art of Dierdre Luzwick.)

# 7

# Treatment Approaches to PTSD

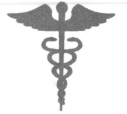

There are many ways to treat post-traumatic stress disorder (PTSD). Most of these treatments interweave and overlap with one another, and many have high success rates in reducing or extinguishing related symptoms and experiences. Sometimes a combination of treatment approaches produces especially positive results. Because each case of PTSD is different, an integrated approach will often provide something of value for those specialists who try it.

When we use the term "treatment approaches" for PTSD, we are referring to systematic programs designed to eliminate or reduce those problematic symptoms and unpleasant experiences associated with an individual's post-traumatic stress. Usually, a qualified person administers these programs to an individual or a group, but some programs are self-administered. All of them are "therapeutic" because they have been designed to promote healing. The word "therapeutic" is derived from the Greek term for a group of professional servants, *therapeutae*. Hence, therapists are specially trained "servants," and therapeutic programs serve people who are in need of help.

Most of these treatment approaches fall under the category of psychotherapy, a program based on psychological principles that is administered by a trained professional practitioner. The goals of these programs include fostering self-understanding and self-acceptance and learning how to change behaviors and beliefs that are harmful because they inhibit a person's enjoyment of life. Almost all psychotherapists are psychologists, psychiatrists, or social workers who have undergone extensive training in order to serve their clients.

But there are also therapeutic programs that are not primarily based on psychological principles. They range from acupuncture to art, from medication to massage. The word "therapy" refers to the remediation or healing of a psychological, physical, or spiritual problem. There are physical therapists, occupational therapists, and speech therapists. In addition, there are spiritual counselors who have been trained to treat spiritual or religious crises, including the loss of one's faith, problems that arise when someone converts from one faith to another, or the difficulties that surface when someone has left a "cult" and attempts to rejoin the larger society.

Some people with PTSD have a religious crisis because a trusted pastor or priest took sexual advantage of them. Other people with PTSD have spiritual crises, such as being plagued with guilt after a good friend was killed in a highway accident when they were driving the car. Religious crises involve aspects of organized religion considered unsavory by the client, while spiritual crises revolve around such topics as one's personal ethics, values, and morals.

Many individual and group approaches are used to treat PTSD. In this chapter, we will describe the most common of these, highlighting those whose effectiveness has been supported by research studies. We usually will use the terms "psychotherapy" and "psychotherapist" when discussing approaches that are based on psychological principles such as memory and learning, and that highlight the relationship between the practitioner and the client. Sometimes, we will utilize the term "talk therapy" when most of the program involves a dialogue between the psychotherapist and the client. Some interventions, such as cognitive-behavior therapy, do not use the term "psychotherapy" and we will honor that preference.

A client is a person who enters psychotherapy; some people prefer the word "patient." However, that term has medical connotations and many treatments for PTSD focus on medication rather than on psychotherapy.

## PSYCHODYNAMIC APPROACHES

The *psychodynamic approach* first emerged in the late 1800s. Sigmund Freud, a physician who lived in Vienna, applied the era's understanding of "energy" to the human psyche. Freud called his approach "psychoanalysis," but it birthed many similar approaches that are now grouped together under the term "psychodynamic psychotherapy." The psychodynamic perspective holds that individuals' problems stem from unconscious conflicts. Conflicting motives and attitudes result in struggles, as people try their best to cope with challenging life experiences, often without much success.

These struggles consume or misdirect one's energy, producing emotional discord. Freud called this energy (or life force) the "libido," and felt it was highly sexual in nature. A person's libido could be blocked by both conscious and unconscious conflicts, usually the latter. These conflicts materialize as symptoms, ranging from backaches to temporary blindness. Freud felt that these symptoms can be removed by psychoanalysis, a type of "talk therapy" in which the psychoanalyst helps a client remove the symptoms—thereby eliminating backaches, restoring sight, and enabling the libidinal energy to flow freely.

Psychoanalysis attempts to trace symptoms back to their origins, sometimes in the form of childhood traumas such as sexual molestation, emotional abuse, sibling rivalry, and dozens of other negative encounters. In the case of what is now called PTSD, Freud attempted to help his clients uncover repressed aspects of the trauma by examining their dreams and "slips of the tongue." He also relied on material that emerged while they were engaged in *free association*—the process of discussing their symptoms and following their own thoughts as they freely associated them with other thoughts and experiences.

Freudian psychoanalysis involves three basic aspects of the human psyche that guide one's psychological development: the *id*, the *ego*, and the *superego*. The id regulates biological drives, motivating individuals to seek pleasure and avoid pain. The superego restrains the id and keeps the life force from flowing too freely by imposing society's moral standards of right and wrong. The ego attempts to balance the drives of the id and the demands of the superego. For example, the id's drive for instant gratification may challenge the superego's demand to postpone pleasure or even deny it if the action does not conform to what society considers "appropriate" behavior. The ego navigates the client through the realities of the world, and Freud's psychoanalytic techniques attempted to endow it with enough energy to help clients function better in their daily lives.

Freud's thoughts about traumatic stress were that it empowers the id, allowing one's biological drives to overpower the logical guidance system of the ego. When this occurs, the superego imposes its own agenda regarding the trauma, evoking shame, guilt, and feelings of inadequacy. According to Freud, when a trauma occurs, the psyche cries out in response to the experience. This pain forces individuals to repress the experience and erect *defense mechanisms* in order to protect themselves against the agony involved in coping with the trauma itself. Examples of these defense mechanisms include avoiding reminders of the trauma or distorting memories of the traumatic experience. But such defenses often inhibit and block the ego's ability to work through the trauma, giving rise to reactions that might seem bizarre. For example, someone may go away from home on the anniversary of a loved one's death, refuse to be a passenger in the type of automobile in which the traumatizing accident occurred, or turn down an invitation to see a particular film because of its similarity to a romantic rejection.

Freudian psychoanalysis is rarely practiced in the United States today because it is a lengthy, time-consuming, and expensive process. However, a variety of psychodynamic psychotherapies are widely used, all of which emphasize the importance of unconscious processes. These psychotherapists might not use such Freudian terms as "libido" or "superego," and may not place as much emphasis as Freud did upon sexuality and unconscious motivation. The therapeutic objective in a psychodynamic approach focuses on building "ego strength," improving self-understanding, and facilitating the capacity to cope, all of which enable individuals to work through and integrate the traumatizing events of their lives (Kudler et al., 2009).

Psychodynamic approaches were found to be effective for many types of disorders in an exhaustive study conducted by Lester Luborsky and his colleagues (1988). Other researchers have found much the same thing, but some of them, including Luborsky, have noted that almost all the major variants of psychotherapy produce similar results.

Psychotherapists who have a psychodynamic orientation see psychotherapy as a gradual process, one consisting of safely encountering and integrating the traumas into the client's present life. This can be challenging, because this type of psychotherapy requires more than insight and reliving traumatic experiences. It is not as long a process as psychoanalysis, which can go on for several years, but is still fairly lengthy, requiring client motivation and what Luborsky called a *therapeutic alliance* between the client and the psychotherapist. This relationship, which is crucial to the success of psychotherapy, usually involves some type of *transference*, in which the client projects parental images and experiences onto the psychotherapist. The resolution of transference issues and the emergence of a client-psychotherapist relationship that is free from distortion are felt to lead to a successful therapeutic outcome. Psychodynamic psychotherapy, at its best, allows change to occur in an atmosphere of trust and safety (Solomon & Johnson, 2002).

Psychodynamic approaches also address such PTSD symptoms as emotional numbing and re-experiencing the trauma in flashbacks and nightmares. Addressing these issues may not be recommended immediately, but may be postponed until sufficient ego strength has been developed.

One of Freud's colleagues, Abram Kardiner, treated hundreds of combat veterans in World War I. Kardiner (1941) published his findings during World War II, accepting Freud's basic premise that psychological trauma was the result of a "breach" in one's psyche. But Kardiner also emphasized the interplay between biological and psychological factors in traumatized combat veterans. The two world wars provided an opportunity for psychodynamic psychotherapy to be applied to what was then referred to as "combat fatigue." The success of these efforts stimulated an interest in psychoanalysis and psychodynamic therapy in the postwar years (Kudler et al., 2009).

Several of Freud's associates, including Alfred Adler, Otto Rank, and Carl Jung, developed their own schools of thought. Adler introduced the terms "sibling rivalry," "lifestyle," and "inferiority complex" into the psychological literature; Rank coined the term "birth trauma," and Jung wrote about "synchronicity," "archetypes," and the "midlife crisis." Somewhat later, the so-called "Neo-Freudians" (or "later Freudians") supplemented Freud's point of view with their own insights. Their number included Karen Horney, Melanie Klein, Harry Stack Sullivan, Erich Fromm, Heinz Hartmann, and Erik Erikson. The Neo-Freudian psychotherapies are grounded in the psychoanalytic concepts of defense mechanisms, unconscious conflicts, transference, and the therapeutic alliance, but they extended the psychodynamic approach into working with couples, groups, and families. Horney, Fromm, and Sullivan could also be called "Neo-Adlerians," because, like Adler, they emphasized power relationships, gender equality, and contemporary social issues.

## COGNITIVE-BEHAVIORAL APPROACHES

Albert Ellis was a U.S. psychologist who originally practiced psychoanalysis. He was especially drawn to the perspective of Alfred Adler because of Adler's emphasis on cognition, or thought processes, and his adherence to the scientific evaluation of psychotherapy. Ellis, feeling that psychoanalysis was too slow and inefficient, started to employ active, directive methods that would work more quickly. He spent less time searching for the unconscious causes of people's problems, preferring to help his clients change those beliefs, attitudes, and behaviors that were blocking their enjoyment of life. In 1957, Ellis published an article comparing his use of psychoanalysis, psychodynamic psychotherapy, and his pioneering "rational psychotherapy," finding the latter to be the most effective. This led to what has become *rational emotive behavior therapy* (REBT), the first of a cascade of cognitive-behavioral approaches that radically altered the psychotherapeutic landscape in the United States and other countries.

The word "behavioral" refers to someone's activities such as the manner in which they relate to other people, the way they perform at work, and how they spend their leisure time during the day. Since all these activities have been learned, REBT focuses on teaching people how to engage in activities that are healthy and satisfying. The word "cognitive" is used to describe a person's thoughts, attitudes, and beliefs, but Ellis used the word "rational" rather than "cognitive" to emphasize the importance of reason, logic, and common sense in making decisions and evaluating one's belief system. At the same time, he also used the term "emotive" to address the importance of emotions and feelings in his work. REBT is a holistic approach that takes into account the inseparable interplay of the client's mind, feelings, and actions.

REBT and other cognitive-behavioral approaches can help people with PTSD change their unhealthy and often harmful personal beliefs. Many of them think and voice such irrational thoughts as, "I do not deserve to recover from my condition; therefore my life is doomed to become one of misery, and that is awful and terrible." Or, "I should have been strong enough to hold back the effects of the trauma, and I am a worthless failure for not doing so." Or, "I did something wrong, and now I am paying for it—stupid wretch that I am."

If individuals plague themselves with such views, then it is necessary for them to deconstruct such harmful beliefs if they want to prevent, lessen, or eliminate PTSD. However, this task is not as easy as it seems as simply identifying irrational beliefs is insufficient. A lasting change in beliefs requires ongoing work, practice, and repetition of the new, rational, and healthy beliefs. Clients who see an REBT psychotherapist are typically given *homework assignments* so that they can vigorously practice putting their new beliefs into action and enjoy the resulting healthier feelings and behaviors.

Albert Ellis and his wife, Debbie Joffe Ellis, wrote about the importance of developing unconditional acceptance of themselves (*unconditional self-acceptance*), of others (*unconditional other acceptance*), and of life itself (*unconditional life acceptance*). Indeed, the philosophy of unconditional acceptance is emphasized more in REBT than in other cognitive-behavioral approaches. According to Ellis and Ellis (2011) unconditional acceptance infuses REBT with compassion and humanism.

Cognitive-behavioral therapists often remark that some of their clients tend to hold onto irrational beliefs despite their restricting nature. Some clients take the position that it is better to live with the unpleasant feelings one knows than to make a change that might bring about new feelings that are even worse. It takes time and commitment to change, especially when—willingly or not—someone is plagued by the horrors of PTSD. If people haunt themselves by continuing to use "self-talk" that is fueled by memories and images of their traumatic experiences, fusing them to the perspective that forms their identity, it is unlikely that they will quickly set aside their old viewpoints and change their perspective. This is particularly true if these individuals are continually reliving the trauma through flashbacks and nightmares. Re-experiencing images of the trauma can bring back the embedded beliefs connected to those experiences.

Cognitive-behavioral schools of thought vary, but typically they include both *psychoeducation* and *stress management skills training*. In psychoeducation, the psychotherapist shares information with clients to help them understand the nature and impact of trauma upon their functioning. It also involves a collaborative search for the cause or causes of their difficulties, emphasizing how their maladaptive behaviors were learned. If they were learned, they can be unlearned, and clients are given a realistic assessment of what they can expect from the course of treatment. These stress management skills almost always include breathing exercises and muscle relaxation. The client learns to breathe slowly and deeply from the diaphragm when feeling stressed and engages in *behavioral rehearsal*, imagining a stressful situation and one's calm and reasoned reaction to it. These skills are useful not only for PTSD survivors, but for others who fall on the traumatic stress spectrum.

Eventually, clients re-imagine the traumatizing event in as much detail as possible. Using *rational emotive imagery*, one of the techniques of REBT, clients vividly imagine the traumatizing event, thus evoking their unhealthy and debilitating emotions. While feeling those emotions, clients deliberately think healthy, rational thoughts to replace the irrational thoughts that contribute to PTSD. In so doing, they change the inept and unhealthy emotions into pleasurable and healthy ones.

Clients also may be asked to provide a number indicating the stress level evoked by the imagined scenario. As the event is imagined over and over again, the stress level generally is lowered. Clients can also be asked to imagine positive ways of dealing with stress in their interactions with other people. This exercise can be followed by a behavioral rehearsal in which the psychotherapist plays the role of someone with whom the client will interact in daily life. The next step is often a homework assignment in which the client actually seeks out a stressful interpersonal interaction and handles it in the healthy way it was rehearsed with the psychotherapist. For example, clients may have been treated badly by people belonging to a particular ethnic group and go out of their way to avoid them. Those clients may be told to find the opportunity to interact with members of that ethnic group to overcome the fear or distaste that was previously associated with such interactions.

Such PTSD symptoms as re-experiencing a trauma are seen as conditioned responses, learned behaviors that need to be unlearned. The futile thoughts and behaviors that people fall into to help them cope with PTSD also need to be unlearned. Avoidance is one example and over-reaction is another—as when a traumatized person lashes out against a member of an ethnic group who has a superficial resemblance to his or her assailant. Neither behavior is useful, adaptive, or rational. However, these behaviors are understandable, and psychoeducation can help clients see the links among early life experiences, the traumatizing event, and what they are telling themselves to evoke, all of which perpetuate the PTSD that followed. Rather than dwelling on the past, cognitive-behavioral therapy emphasizes the client's present state of affairs and a future that can be better through the tools of REBT and similar approaches. A few of these approaches will now be described.

### Cognitive Behavioral Therapy (CBT)

Aaron Beck (1976) developed *cognitive therapy* to treat depression, an approach that eventually morphed into what the books of his daughter, Judith Beck (2011), refer to as *cognitive behavioral therapy* (CBT). As Ellis first did in the 1950s, the Becks point out that the interpretation of an event, rather than the event itself, is what determines an emotional reaction. Ellis frequently cited the ancient Greek philosopher, Epictetus, who had written much the same thing two thousand years earlier. As you know by now, we have made distinctions between potentially traumatizing events, traumatizing events, and traumatic experiences. An event can be traumatizing for one person, but not for another because they experience it differently as a result of their beliefs, personal myths, and worldviews.

CBT psychotherapists work with their clients to test the usefulness of their thoughts, perceptions, and attitudes in everyday life. Some of these cognitions often are found to be negative and harmful. For example, a client may overgeneralize, blame other people for his or her misfortunes, or view the world in terms of "right" and "wrong" with no middle ground. The cognitive-behavioral therapist and client work together, finding alternative explanations and beliefs. This is often followed by homework assignments to put these alternatives into practice. As a result, the client learns and practices new cognitions by adopting new, and potentially more fulfilling, behaviors.

In applying CBT to PTSD survivors, the psychotherapist might encourage self-talk (in which clients talk to themselves about problems and their solutions), design self-training around dysfunctional beliefs and habits, assign tasks to carry out at home (homework), and shift a client's perspective of the traumatic experiences. This shift of perspective is called *reframing*, or putting something into a different framework or worldview. These techniques and others like them create the possibility for clients to learn, adapt, and abandon irrational, harmful thoughts and beliefs along with behaviors that prevent personal growth. Clients can then begin to relate to this new framework as they develop new beliefs and behaviors.

There are many variations of CBT. *Stress inoculation therapy* is unique because it provides clients with skills to handle stressful situations. For example, Martha told her husband that she was "stressed out" at work because her supervisor was constantly putting her down and criticizing her. Martha did not dare complain about his treatment of her, because he had a position of considerable power in the company. Martha began to have frightening nightmares in which her supervisor chastised her in a loud voice, holding a whip that he used to underscore his criticisms. Martha's husband suggested that she reframe the situation, using it as an example of sexism in the workplace. He suggested that she keep a notebook and record each instance of harassment. He further suggested that she write the words "On the Job Abuse" in her notebook and record the "Abuse of the Day." Martha took his advice, and soon her fellow workers saw the notebook and wanted to read its contents. When this news reached the supervisor, he became extremely embarrassed, knowing that, if Martha's notebook was made public, his job would be in jeopardy. Soon the harassment stopped, but Martha kept her notebook in her desk and made sure that her supervisor knew about it!

### Acceptance and Commitment Therapy (ACT)

*Acceptance and commitment therapy* (ACT) uses reframing to help clients increase awareness and acknowledgment of their beliefs associated with the trauma. ACT focuses on a client's attempts to avoid reliving traumatic experiences.

By putting considerable effort into avoidance, the clients actually increase their proclivity to re-experience the trauma. When this occurs, they often take drastic steps to avoid reliving the traumatic experiences by engaging in substance abuse. When this group of traumatized people turns to alcohol, they obtain temporary relief from their symptoms. In the play *Cat on a Hot Tin Roof*, the traumatized Brick tells Maggie, his wife, that he drinks and drinks and drinks until there is a "click" in his mind; at that moment, he has found peace. Once he becomes sober, he needs to start the process over again, because the urge to avoid the trauma emerges anew.

Once clients understand that the thoughts, beliefs, and emotions related to their trauma are not a central part of their personal identity, they can safely review and relive the traumatic experience. If Brick had seen a cognitive-behavioral psychotherapist, he would have been a much happier person, and his wife Maggie would not have been so sexually frustrated. But then, the ensuing play would have not been worth writing, producing, or staging! A cat resting comfortably on a pillow is not as theatrically exciting as a cat on a hot tin roof, scampering to avoid the pain.

As clients begin to understand that what they believe impacts their functioning, an opportunity occurs for them to change their behavior. Psychotherapy helps clients gain greater clarity about their lives and explore new beliefs and changes in behavior. Accepting their internal experiences and increasing the awareness and understanding of their beliefs is only one psychotherapeutic goal. To improve their quality of life, clients need to work through life transitions and responsibilities. For example, if certain relationships are no longer satisfying, whether they be with a spouse, partner, friend, or a colleague at work, adjustments need to be made, if possible. This process often entails finding new work or "breaking" from a particular relationship.

It is not enough to simply "move on" and hope that any dysfunctional routines will subside. Transitioning is healthy, but if behaviors are not confronted they will most likely reoccur. As a result, in ACT and other types of cognitive-behavioral therapy, responsibility is placed on the client to be proactive in working to change behaviors, while the therapist assists the client to find direction and understanding.

Applying these therapeutic concepts requires that cognitive-behavioral therapists help their clients modify those beliefs that are not rational, useful, or practical. This allows clients to understand how their thought and behavior patterns served to protect them from the trauma, while failing to support healthy living in the present moment.

### Exposure Therapy (EX)

Like ACT, a key goal of *exposure therapy* (EX) is the clients' acceptance of their traumatic experiences as a prelude to draining them of their emotional impact. Exposure therapy attempts this by confronting clients with stimuli associated with the trauma in their lives or in their imagination. This is done repeatedly until the negative emotions have been extinguished. EX often begins by exposing clients to the element of the trauma that rates highest on their *anxiety hierarchy*, or in some cases, on the element that rates lowest. This decision depends on the psychotherapist and on the sensitivity of the client. In psychodynamic psychotherapy, the most disturbing aspects of PTSD are dealt with later in treatment, but in ACT and EX they might be attacked early in the treatment. In any event, clients are repeatedly exposed to frightening stimuli until their anxiety diminishes and the escape and avoidance behavior ceases.

There are several ways that clients' confrontation with their traumatic experiences can take place. A client can discuss the trauma, in the present tense, repeatedly and in detail. A psychotherapist may also provide a scenario, based on knowledge of the event, while the client listens. A psychotherapeutic session can provide exposure, along with relaxation exercises or psychoeducation, in which the client's destructive beliefs about the traumatizing event are discussed and dispelled. This repetition is often called "flooding," and the end result is termed "habituation." A variant is *prolonged exposure therapy* in which mental imagery is used extensively. Whenever possible, a direct experience of the situation associated with the traumatizing event is also provided (Foa et al., 2007). Most mental imagery exercises involve visual images, since the visual-motor cortex resides near many of the brain's emotional regulation centers. Imagery rehearsal is a key component of many CBTs, as vivid images can activate the same brain centers that are involved in the actual behavior once it is initiated.

Another variant is *virtual reality exposure therapy* (VRET) in which sounds, smells, and sights (sometimes in 3-D) that correspond with the traumatizing event are included. For example, as a combat veteran, wearing goggles over the eyes, begins to recall a traumatizing incident, a clinician introduces appropriate elements into the environment. A car bomb suddenly explodes, a building catches fire, and a sniper unleashes a volley of bullets. Other simulated sights and sounds might include rockets, gunfire, and babies crying. The guiding concept of VRET is to gradually reintroduce veterans to the events that triggered their trauma until the memory no longer incapacitates them (Wiederhold & Wiederhold, 2004). "Full Spectrum Warrior" is one of many packaged scenarios available for applying VRET in work with combat veterans. Another scenario, "Virtual Iraq" is customized for veterans returning from Iraq with PTSD.

EX, like all cognitive-behavioral approaches, incorporates *learning theory*—what is known about the way people learn. This group of approaches focuses on learning new ways of thinking and behaving while trying not to access one's unconscious to find the "cause" of a symptom. Instead of becoming "trauma junkies" who dwell incessantly on the causes of their trauma, clients are taught how to desensitize themselves to the trauma (Abramowitz, Deacon, & Whiteside, 2011).

### Cognitive Processing Therapy (CPT)

CPT includes elements of exposure therapy, but places its major emphasis upon examining and changing the client's belief system. The CPT psychotherapist challenges those beliefs that are problematic, attempts to unravel traumatic experiences, and works to undo such emotional patterns as self-blame and undeserved guilt.

In this approach, clients write a detailed account of their traumatic experiences and then read the account to the psychotherapist. This narrative is used to uncover the points where the client is stuck and unable to move, as well as the beliefs that are particularly difficult to change. These "stuck points" become the focus of processing in CPT and receive considerable attention. Originally designed for group work with women who had been raped, CPT has been applied to other PTSD groups as well (Cahill et al., 2009, p. 199).

### Dialectical Behavioral Therapy (DBT)

A "dialectical" approach to psychotherapy emphasizes the back-and-forth dialogue between a "thesis," or habitual way of thinking and feeling, and an "antithesis," a radically new way of being. For a *dialectical behavioral therapy* (DBT) client, the thesis is the resistance to change and the antithesis is the need to enter psychotherapy. The best possible outcome would be a "synthesis," where clients give up their detrimental behaviors and build upon their strengths, while adding new skills as a result of DBT. Advocates of DBT point out an additional dialectic between biological and environmental factors—that is, some clients may be extremely sensitive due to their biology, but have learned to manage their emotional reactions so they do not become a handicap. Others may be biologically predisposed to have what some psychologists call "thin boundaries" and become susceptible to traumatizing events. The first group of people, those with "thick boundaries," may be less likely to develop PTSD than their "thin-boundary" neighbors.

Feinstein and Krippner (2008) have used the dialectical approach to help people improve their *personal mythologies* or worldviews. When an individual's "old myth" (or thesis) is found wanting, one may shift to a "counter-myth" (or antithesis) that is drastically different but impractical. Eventually, a "new myth" evolves that is a synthesis of the best of both worldviews. A PTSD client may refuse to discuss a traumatizing event with anyone such as being scolded by an emotionally abusive parent until the pent-up pressure produces a reaction. This reaction, or antithesis, may result in a compulsion to talk about the insults, put-downs, and name-callings with anyone who will listen. Needless to say, this behavior is not likely to win friends or influence people. Following psychotherapy, a synthesis is reached where memories of the abuse will be selectively discussed with close friends at appropriate times.

Feinstein and Krippner's (2008) workbook contains many exercises that had their roots in REBT and other cognitive-behavioral approaches to psychotherapy. One exercise asks clients to identify an emotional wound (an old myth) that resists healing. In their imagination, the clients come up with a new direction (a counter-myth), but one that is unrealistic. The two myths engage in a back-and-forth argument, or dialectic, until a realistic, practical direction is discovered. The new myth is then translated into behaviors that the clients can implement into their daily lives. This exercise resembles a CBT technique in which clients write a detailed account of the trauma and read it back to the therapist in an attempt to discover "stuck points," or times during the incident that evoked conflict with previously held beliefs. These points receive particular attention during therapy, and the clients are encouraged to challenge such problematic beliefs as blaming themselves for the trauma (McCann & Pearlman, 1990). One's beliefs about safety, trust, power, control, intimacy, and self-acceptance are what Feinstein and Krippner would call personal myths, and a dialectical approach can often lead to a resolution.

## HUMANISTIC AND EXISTENTIAL APPROACHES

Since PTSD survivors are often struggling to construct something meaningful from their experiences, no amount of superficial work can relieve their deep conflicts. Clients often ask, "Why did this happen to me?" and "What does this all mean?" The self-talk of psychodynamic psychotherapy and the desensitization of cognitive-behavioral approaches may bypass these core issues. Clients suffering from self-isolation, interpersonal detachment, and the conviction that their world is no longer safe often require special attention. Practitioners of *humanistic and existential psychotherapy* believe that their approaches are uniquely equipped to provide the answers. Carl Jung once remarked, "I am not what happened to me. I am what I choose to become." This statement nicely discriminates between a traumatizing event and the subsequent traumatic experience, while also striking an existential note in its emphasis on the importance of choice.

Both humanistic psychology and existential psychology assume that human beings have some ability to choose and to take responsibility for their choices. Furthermore, humans are considered to be *intentional* and tend to move toward goals, consciously or unconsciously. They seek to bring meaning, value, and creativity into their lives, even when their attempts are irrational, dysfunctional, and impractical. The psychotherapist attempts to establish an alliance with the client in which intentions can be clarified and activated.

Existential psychology, which originated in Europe, is associated with the existential school of philosophy. It attracted the attention of the U.S. psychotherapist Rollo May, who was among those who brought it to the United States. Humanistic psychology, which originated in the United States, spans a wide range of psychotherapies including Carl Rogers's *person-centered approach*. Albert Ellis considered REBT to be humanistic as well as cognitive-behavioral, even though his very direct style of helping people confront their irrational beliefs dramatically contrasted with Carl Rogers's indirect style.

Victor Frankl, an Austrian psychiatrist, spent three years in a Nazi concentration camp due to his Jewish heritage. Instead of giving in to depression, he used his experiences to develop *logotherapy*, one of the first existential psychotherapies. Charlotte Bühler was a German psychologist and psychotherapist who moved to the United States in 1938, knowing that if she stayed in Europe she would end up in a concentration camp because of her Jewish background. Bühler brought her knowledge of child development to humanistic psychology, becoming a central figure in the movement. James Bugental exemplified a practitioner who expertly combined humanistic and existential psychotherapy into an elegant system. Yet not all of these pioneers were psychotherapists: psychologists Abraham Maslow and Anthony Sutich, who founded *The Journal of Humanistic Psychology* in 1961, advocated an exploration of the depths and the heights of human nature as well as the alterations in consciousness that could be used to foster human potential.

### Humanistic-Existential Psychotherapy

From the humanistic-existential perspective, cognitive-behavioral approaches suffice as band-aid interventions to help PTSD survivors cope with their symptoms. As a result, they often fail to help clients work through the catastrophic impacts the traumatic experiences have had upon their way of *being in the world*, as the existentialists would phrase it. Helping PTSD survivors understand who they are and how they can operate in a world that may seem suddenly foreign requires a reorganization of their personal identity, self-concepts, and worldviews. Humanistic-existential approaches attempt to help clients grapple with the basic nature and meaning of their experiences, whether positive or negative.

Here is an example. Anne was a star basketball player in high school and was a member of her college team as well. One night she accepted a ride home from a party with three male students. They stopped at their own apartment and proceeded to rape her. Anne's fury increased, when her assailants, all sports stars at the college, merely received short-term suspensions from school and were not prosecuted. Anne developed an aversion to parties, to basketball, and to anything else that reminded her of the traumatizing event. Some of her classmates suspected that what Anne called a "gang rape" was actually an "orgy," because all the participants, including Anne, had been drinking. Anne's anger increased and she began seeing a psychotherapist, who allowed Anne to do most of the talking, following Rogers's person-centered approach. Anne told her story many times and began to consider transferring to another school, one in which there would be no reminders of her assault. Once she followed through with this decision, her symptoms began to abate.

Anne's therapist employed humanistic-existential methods, because he believed that people are *self-actualizing* and thus, are capable of making resourceful and beneficial changes in their lives. Like Alfred Adler, humanistic-existential psychotherapists understand that clients live in a social-historical context, and that their choices shape how they encounter present and future circumstances. For example, Anne's psychotherapist helped her to understand why her assailants received relatively light punishments—the college needed their skills to enhance its reputation in the field of basketball. A championship team can draw favorable attention that will attract new students and additional money. This state of affairs was neither fair nor just, but Anne began to realize that she lives in a world whether fairness and justice are rare commodities.

Martin Buber was an existential philosopher who wrote about the "I-Thou" relationship and how it allows for greater intimacy than the "I-It" relationship. The "deep work" with a PTSD client begins by building a supportive therapeutic alliance between the therapist and client. This "I-Thou" relationship is the crux of humanistic-existential psychotherapy; if no connection or bond develops between the client and the therapist, psychotherapy may be ineffective. Development of this type of relationship is a difficult feat for PTSD survivors. Trust, an important quality from the client's viewpoint, has been scarred or broken, thus provoking many clients to avoid exposing their vulnerability. As a result, the importance of establishing this bond cannot be overestimated. The time it takes to create a trusting relationship is often fraught with *boundary testing* with the psychotherapist. If the psychotherapist is perceived as untrustworthy, then the potential for change is diminished.

Once a trusting relationship has been initiated, humanistic-existential psychotherapists employ several methods for deep life-changing work. They try to help clients feel their worthiness, understand their personal mythologies, make sense of what might seem senseless, while creating and refining their potential strengths and talents. The humanistic-existential approach does not view clients as machines to be "fixed," or even as people who need to "adjust" to their world. Instead, psychotherapy is viewed as a collaborative and creative process that helps clients to look within themselves for the resources that will help them recover from their trauma. In this way, humanistic-existential psychotherapists acknowledge their clients' needs to integrate their traumatic experiences into the rest of their lives and strive toward making meaning of them in the present context.

The goal of humanistic-existential psychotherapy is to empower clients, helping them to realize that they can value and enjoy a self-guided, authentic life as they really are, instead of who they think they should be. Psychotherapy helps clients nurture ignored or neglected capacities as well as to recognize the influences both from inside themselves and from their environments. Among these explorations in humanistic-existential psychotherapy, especially when working with PTSD survivors, is the area of religion and spirituality. Clients need to be encouraged to explore their own connection to what they consider "sacred" and "divine," and the psychotherapist needs to provide the necessary "space" for such a quest.

Oftentimes, a psychotherapist's own biases can emerge in the midst of the client's discovery. Hence, it is important that psychotherapists understand their own belief systems and worldviews, along with their personal experiences that can help facilitate a discussion. Because one's spiritual convictions are often challenged by traumatic experiences, it comes as no surprise that religious practitioners are among the first to see individuals after they have encountered a trauma. Often, traumatic experiences can challenge individuals' beliefs about death, identity, isolation, and other important concerns. Influenced by the writings of Otto Rank, a group of existentially-oriented psychologists has developed "Terror Management Theory," which holds that one's terror in the face of inevitable death is a primary motivator of human activities. Many people with PTSD have faced the threat of death directly, whether on the battlefield, in a motor vehicle accident, being held for ransom, or being caught in an avalanche. Attempting to navigate through life may be difficult when the experiences of trauma are compounding the meaning-making activities that are a part of everyday challenges in the 21st century.

### Positive Psychology

The practice of *positive psychology* (Seligman & Csikszentmihalyi, 2000) has its roots in Abraham Maslow's emphasis on human potentials, in contrast to psychoanalysis' focus on human frailties and negative experiences. In fact, Maslow coined the term "positive psychology" in 1970. Following Maslow's lead, positive psychologists attempt to identify and strengthen the healthy capabilities of people, believing that they can be taught positive attitudes, *learned optimism* being one of them, and *authentic happiness* another.

Positive psychologists assert that their studies are conducted within the framework of mainstream science, while maintaining that humanistic-existential approaches have failed to rigorously study the outcomes of the counseling and psychotherapy they provide. Humanistic-existential psychologists, in response, contend that their approaches always have been and continue to be grounded in empirical quantitative and qualitative research (Elliot & Greenberg, 2001). Also, humanistic-existential psychotherapists score positive psychology's inability to sufficiently recognize the often valuable functions played in a person's growth by such "negative" emotions as anger, sorrow, and fear. Positive psychology has been criticized for alleged slick marketing and for disregarding harsh and unforgiving societal realities such as poverty and warfare. Nevertheless, positive psychology has organized a number of research programs for the study of human capacities and has attracted favorable attention from people who had previously dismissed other schools of psychology because of their apparent emphasis on pathology.

### Transpersonal Psychology

*Transpersonal psychology* is also rooted in the work of Abraham Maslow. He and his colleague Anthony Sutich founded *The Journal of Transpersonal Psychology* in 1969, a move that launched transpersonal psychology into the realms of important fields of study. If *psychology* can be defined as the scientific study of experience and behavior, then *transpersonal psychology* studies those experiences and behaviors in which people seem to transcend their ordinary self-identity. This can be done either spontaneously, through the use of such contemplative disciplines as prayer and meditation, through such active disciplines as yoga or the martial arts, or through the use of mind-altering plants and chemicals including peyote, "psychedelic" mushrooms, ayahuasca (a tea made from plants found in the Amazon valley), LSD, mescaline, or psilocybin. Each of these practices can be utilized in psychotherapy with a PTSD survivor, either as the main approach or as a supplement to psychodynamic, cognitive-behavioral, or humanistic-existential psychotherapy.

Transpersonal psychotherapy often incorporates a client's religious convictions, a topic that Carl Jung took seriously despite its dismissal by Freud and Adler. Such organized religious or philosophical systems as Taoism, Buddhism, Islam, Christianity, and Hinduism, as well as one's own belief structures, find a niche in transpersonal psychotherapy. However, people with a PTSD diagnosis who consider themselves "spiritual," as opposed to "religious," may also be attracted to the transpersonal perspective. A "religious" person operates from the standpoint of an organized religion such as Judaism or Roman Catholicism, while the "spiritual" person venerates God, Nature, the Tao, or some other benevolent entity, attempting to lead a moral and ethical life outside of an organized body of "believers" who adhere to a particular belief system or dogma. Both perspectives are often ignored by other psychotherapeutic approaches, but their orientation is an important element in humanistic-existential and transpersonal psychotherapies.

The field of psychotherapy is not limited to clinical psychologists, psychiatrists, and psychiatric social workers. Adequately trained counselors, spiritual advisors, and other mental health professionals often work with PTSD. However, one survey discovered that only one of out five mental health practitioners of any background or orientation had been trained to work in the area of PTSD. Therefore, practitioners of transpersonal psychotherapy have a unique advantage in possessing skills that their colleagues with other backgrounds lack. At the same time, they must also have obtained the information and skills that allow them to "do no harm," as Hippocrates admonished centuries ago. Poorly executed interventions with PTSD survivors can do more harm than good, even re-traumatizing the client or making it unlikely that a second "shrink" will ever be consulted.

### Relational Dharma

Trauma often has an immediate impact. The disruption of a person's balance can result in a "shattering" that can lead to the destruction of one's self-regulation capacities or even to a break in the flow of life experience, such as noted in our previous discussion of dissociation. As an approach to the resolution of trauma, Relational Dharma (RD) supports a holistic reintegration of the traumatized individual's experience, as it is encountered within the *intersubjective* field between the client and psychotherapist (or other RD-trained health care provider). The term "intersubjectivity" refers to the factors that connect two separate psyches. It is conventionally used within the fields of philosophy and psychology as a means to illustrate reciprocal developmental influences made accessible by the relationship shared between two individuals. In this way, the intersubjective space provides the context for a reciprocal formation to develop between the RD practitioner and the trauma survivor, propelling an opportunity for a new understanding and vision of oneself to emerge.

Relational Dharma, developed by psychologist Jeannine Davies (2011), puts forth a transformational model and psychotherapeutic path of intersubjectivity. This process involves a progressive realization of human nature as an interdependent and inseparable unity, which is discovered through insight into the bond of human interrelatedness. From this understanding, higher forms of relatedness are both discovered and fostered. In turn, this promotes greater forms of freedom, both for oneself and in relationship with others.

Examples of these forms of freedom expressed through *higher human relatedness* (HHR) include the inner liberty to feel another's suffering as inseparable to one's own and the compassion to seek to alleviate it, thus respecting the freedom of others as inseparable to one's own freedom. Another expression of HHR is the freedom to forgive others for their transgressions. In order to forgive, the ability to "step back" and recognize the conditions that gave rise to his or her actions versus reacting from a place of personalizing these actions, must be developed. As awareness into the causal relationships that led this person to act in a harmful way becomes recognized, relational objectivity emerges and compassion becomes possible. This understanding can be a known as the *dharma*, the principles governing liberation from fear, aggression, and ignorance as well as the principles elevating courage, kindness, and the wisdom that recognizes life's inherent unity. Since these principles or *dharmas* are universal, and are understood in context to the relational structures and forms governing human suffering and human freedom within intersubjectivity, the term "Relational Dharma" is used.

Relational Dharma's core framework is a contemporary re-envisioning of the central teaching of Buddhism of the interdependence of all life. RD holds that insight into interdependence can be gained through human relationship, which, in turn, supports the emergence of HHR. It is in this way that the progression of insight within RD then becomes the bridge between people. This bridge helps to expand each individual's own nature and advance HHR, such as the capacity for forgiveness.

Utilizing the immediacy of the encounter between the RD practitioner and the PTSD survivor, the Relational Dharma approach creates the possibility of transforming negative or life-diminishing "filters" into associations that widen and deepen identity. The appearance of something "foreign," "not part of," or "too much," is relaxed, so that one's sense of what constitutes a "whole person" naturally broadens and evolves. But the process does not end there; it goes on to include a deeper understanding of the relationship between oneself and others. In this way, RD becomes a means toward a simultaneous release from the trauma that evoked the experience of suffering. There is also a release from the PTSD survivor's identification with earlier negatively conditioned behaviors and experiences.

From this new orientation, expressions of higher human relatedness naturally emerge which, in turn, promote greater freedom to oneself and in relationship to others. In the case of the PTSD survivor, he or she may find the freedom to release from the isolation and imprisonment of living in hatred toward their oppressor. Instead, he or she, in recognition of the deep interdependence of human life, can choose to become a "voice for the voiceless," someone who seeks to bring peace to all victims, the oppressor and oppressed alike.

Chinese dissidents are examples of this phenomenon. Wei Jingsheng took part in the "democracy wall" movement in 1978, posting calls for democracy on a special wall reserved for "free speech." When the democracy wall attracted undue attention, Wei was sentenced to solitary confinement for two decades. Once Wei was released, he left the country but discovered that his ability to work was inhibited by crippling rage. It is this emotional reaction that needs to be released before Wei and those like him can become effective voices for their cause.

## MIND-BODY APPROACHES

*Mind-body approaches* use thoughts and emotions to influence the physical symptoms of PTSD. The ancient Greek physician Hippocrates wrote, "The natural healing force within each of us is the greatest force in getting well." This is the goal of each of the mind-body approaches. Traditional Chinese, Japanese, and Indian medicine emphasizes the links between mind and body, but, until recently, Western medicine kept the two systems separate. However, in the 1960s, Herbert Benson, a physician, began treating stressed-out people with the *relaxation response*, an adaptation of various meditation programs. About the same time, the psychiatrist George Solomon observed that rheumatoid arthritis got worse when people were depressed. He discovered links between emotions and the immune system, naming this new field of *psychoneuroimmunology*, or PNI. When the study of the endocrine system was added to the study of psychology and neurology, the term "psychoneuroendocrinology" was sometimes used, but PNI practitioners normally include in their work such endocrine glands as the pituitary, thyroid, and gonads and the hormones they secrete.

During that same period, Robert Ader, a psychologist, discovered that rats could learn how to change the responses of their immune system, even though it had been assumed that there was no connection between the nervous system and the immune system. Ader even found that the immunology of ailing rats could be improved through conditioning, whenever their caretaker entered the room. Candice Pert, a pharmacologist, investigated neuropeptides and neurotransmitters, often referred to as "messenger cells." She described a network of "emotion molecules" that included the brain, the gut, and other parts of the body.

All of these pioneers spearheaded mind-body approaches to medicine and psychotherapy, the common thread being that people were able to exert voluntary control over bodily functions to a degree previously thought impossible. Traumatic experiences release stress hormones that can affect the immune system, increasing people's vulnerability to illness. Mind-body approaches attempt to reduce the level of stress hormones in the body so that the immune system is better equipped to repel sickness (Vitetta et al., 2005).

### Biofeedback and Neurofeedback

In *biofeedback*, an external monitoring device that provides clients with information regarding their biological states often enables them to exert voluntary control over blood pressure, heart rate, and other involuntary functions once thought to be resistant to learning. The term "neurofeedback" is used when the learning strategy involves the control of brain waves to reduce headaches and hypertension. In both biofeedback and neurofeedback, bodily functioning is revealed through a video display or an auditory signal. For example, clients with PTSD may attempt to change the color of the display or lower the tone of the signal to reduce their stress levels.

Biofeedback and neurofeedback have been used to treat combat veterans, resulting in an increase of interpersonal skills and positive feelings along with decreased anxiety, hostility, and panic. In one study, U.S. Marine and Navy veterans were enrolled in a program that combined biofeedback and neurofeedback with cognitive, resilience, and relationship retraining, as well as virtual reality exposure therapy. One of the positive outcomes of this program was a decrease in heart rate irregularities. (One's heartbeat is controlled by the autonomic nervous system, once thought to be resistant to voluntary manipulation.)

## Meditation

There are many types of meditation, but all of them assist clients to voluntarily control their attention, helping them to live in the present, rather than being preoccupied with past errors and future apprehensions. Originally a spiritual discipline, meditation can be utilized with or without a devotional, transcendental aspect. *Mindfulness meditation* asks clients to focus their attention on their moment-by-moment thoughts and sensations. "Mindful" clients learn how to enjoy each bite of food, each color in a sunset, and each tone of a bell or a chant, making it less likely that they will engage in re-experiencing a trauma. In *transcendental meditation*, clients repeat a *mantra* (a single word or phrase) continuously several times each day. It is one form of *concentrative meditation* in which clients focus on a single stimulus; besides the mantra, it can be a *yantra* (or image) or a thought. *Insight meditation* (or *Vipassana*) emphasizes self-observation and introspection, thereby revealing how the mind was disturbed and what needs to be done to keep it from being disturbed again.

Both neurofeedback and meditation can help the brain deal with an environment that most PTSD clients find over-stimulating. One way they do this is to increase the number of *alpha waves* produced by the brain and decrease the number of *beta waves*. The latter brain waves characterize rapid thought, while alpha waves are much slower and help "turn down the volume" on distracting information. After an eight-week mindfulness meditation program sponsored by Harvard Medical School, people who had never meditated before were able to learn how to be "mindful," increase their attention span, and decrease their perception of pain.

The stereotyped picture of a meditator is of someone who is sitting peacefully. However, there are many types of movement meditations, especially those that originated in the *martial arts*, a collection of tactics for self-defense or offense, as the occasion demands. *Tai chi chuan* is the most popular form of exercise on the planet. It started out as a martial art, but has morphed into a technique for maintaining and improving one's health. It combines deep breathing with intricate movements that require its practitioners to not let their minds wander to other topics. Many of its movements are named after animals and birds, reflecting its origins in ancient Chinese shamanism. Such titles as "white crane" and "crouching tiger" are reminiscent of the shamans' connection with Nature and their claims to "shape shift," transforming themselves into an animal or bird.

*Qigong* also is associated with shamanism as well as with traditional Chinese medicine. It is used as a meditative practice in both the Buddhist and Taoist spiritual traditions. Meditative training in Qigong utilizes mantras, yantras, deep breathing, and bodily postures. The central focus in Qigong is the regulation, control, and manipulation of *qi*, a form of "life energy." According to both the Buddhist and Taoist philosophies, *qi* needs to be regulated through three inter-connected components: the mind, the body, and the spirit. Followers of Confucius use Qigong meditation for the purpose of enlightenment and the development of virtue.

*Yoga* is associated with meditative practices in Hinduism, Buddhism, and Jainism. Originating in India, yoga has several branches including *hatha yoga*, *karma yoga*, *kundalini yoga*, and *raja yoga*. The Indian seer Patanjali is widely regarded as the founder of formal yoga philosophy, principally raja yoga, defined as a system for the control of the mind. Patanjali advocated a seated position for meditation, controlled breathing or *pranayama*, and fixing attention on an object in an attempt to "merge" with it. Centuries later, a series of *asanas*, or postures, were developed that are associated with yoga today. Again, many of them are given such names as "cobra," linking them with the energizing forces of Nature.

*Kundalini yoga* is based on what is called the "coiled snake" at the base of the spine; with discipline, it can gradually "uncoil," bringing *enlightenment* to the practitioner. Premature "kundalini awakening" can become what many transpersonal psychologists refer to as a "spiritual emergency" one that requires careful treatment by a spiritual practitioner rather than medical intervention. Zen Buddhist meditation has some of its roots in yogic practices, and yoga is central to Tibetan Buddhism and to the Jain spiritual tradition. *Tantra* is an esoteric form of both Hinduism and Buddhism, one that employs yogic practices emphasizing *mudras*, or stylized gestures, and *mandalas*, or symbolic drawings. "Left-handed" tantra is celebrated for its inclusion of disciplined sexual intercourse in its rituals, but most forms of tantra are content to obtain "bliss" through the breathing exercises. Sexual difficulties accompany many cases of PTSD (including 80% of PTSD in combat veterans), hence "left-handed" tantra might deserve more respect and consideration than it has received.

Any of these meditative practices are of potential use to PTSD survivors. By paying attention to present activities, one is less likely to dwell on past traumas. In addition, such martial arts as *Aikido, Kung Fu, Jiu-Jitsu, Teikwondo, Angolan Capoeira,* and *Brazilian Capoeira* can serve as a healthy outlet for feelings of anger and aggression as well as a means of engaging in group activities. Mainstream team sports such as basketball, football, and soccer can do the same. And for those who are suspicious of "Eastern" rituals, various Christian, Jewish, and Muslim congregations have advocated prayer instead of meditation, and have permitted the practice of yoga if it is stripped of its spiritual elements and used only as a physical exercise.

### Hypnosis

There are several approaches to *clinical hypnosis*, but they all involve a practitioner, usually referred to as a "hypnotist," who suggests that a client experience changes in perception, cognition, emotion, or behavior. Sometimes these suggestions are direct, but sometimes they are indirect, and sometimes the suggestions are initiated by the clients. This latter procedure is referred to as *self-hypnosis*.

People vary in their responsiveness to suggestion, but it can be a valuable human potential. The roles of expectancy, hope, and faith are emphasized in clinical hypnosis. The rationale for treating trauma through hypnosis was originally described by the French psychiatrist Pierre Janet in 1924, but there were no formal studies until 2008. Israeli practitioners assigned 32 veterans who were already in treatment into two groups. One group was given Zopidem, a medication, while members of the other group were hypnotized, using a program geared to alleviate their symptoms. The hypnosis group fared much better than the Zopidem group, especially with regard to their quality of sleep, the alleviation of their depression, and their ability to concentrate. One month later, all of these improvements were still in place.

Hypnosis also has been used in conjunction with *exposure response prevention therapy*, a cognitive-behavioral treatment that consists of an actual confrontation with an actual or imagined fear stimulus. The therapist and the client create a "fear hierarchy," noting the objects and experiences that are least and most feared. First, the therapist demonstrates how the client may react in a rational way during the exposure, for example, to a loud noise or a suspicious-looking stranger. Then, the client follows the example, performing this ritual several times while hypnotized. Eventually, the client is able to confront the fear without hypnosis and carry what has been learned into daily life. You may recall the anxiety hierarchy described above in the context of exposure therapy; a similar continuum can be constructed for fear and used as a preventive measure.

### Relaxation

Doesn't relaxation come easily? Why does someone have to be taught to relax? People with PTSD tend to be "on guard" most of the time. Even when they try to relax, a part of them is afraid to lose control. As a result, they sacrifice calmness for tension, tranquility for perpetual apprehension. One of the most popular relaxation techniques is *autogenic training,* in which the client is taught to combine mental imagery with slow breathing and attention to body sensations. For example, the client can imagine being at a tropical beach, breathing easily, while his or her arms are sinking into the sand. Attention can be paid to a regular heartbeat, a cool forehead, and a warm tummy. Once they have learned this procedure from a practitioner, clients can carry out this program themselves.

*Progressive relaxation* focuses on the body's muscles, beginning with the toes and working toward the head. The client becomes aware of any tension that exists and then increases that tension. This is followed by total relaxation, and the client is taught to observe the difference. Each of the major muscle groups is tensed, and then relaxed, unwinding the client's muscle groups, one at a time. As is the case with autogenic training, clients can learn how to self-administer this routine.

Relaxation can also be attained through self-hypnosis, mindfulness meditation, the martial arts, the relaxation response, and many other mind-body approaches. People with PTSD tend to be physically and emotionally stressed. Their bodies release stress hormones that have negative effects on health in general. Stress that is related to anger and anxiety can affect the heart and immune system. Stress that is related to depression can diminish any number of body functions. The goal of relaxation approaches is to encourage the body and mind to relax, helping the immune system to fight off illness and initiate healing. In addition to PTSD, relaxation can have a positive effect on asthma, obesity, stomach and intestinal problems, insomnia, and such menopausal symptoms as "hot flashes" and depression.

### Energy Psychology

Traditional Chinese medicine treats a loss or imbalance of *body energies* called *qi* with acupuncture, diet, massage, and herbs. A number of practitioners have adapted these practices into a variety of approaches under the umbrella term of *energy psychology* (EP). Many EP practitioners claim to have treated PTSD successfully by combining mental imagery, verbal affirmations, and the stimulation of acupuncture points, or, in some cases, with the *chakras*—the hypothetical energy centers of Indian Ayurvedic medicine.

The use of EP can be demonstrated with the case of Rich (Paulson & Krippner, 2007, pp. 122–123). Rich was hospitalized, disabled by insomnia, haunted by combat memories, and terrified by heights, a residue of his parachute jumps. During treatment, he was asked to imagine a situation involving heights, whereupon his fear level increased immediately. While holding a mental image of this event, Rich was asked to tap certain points on his skin. Within a few minutes, Rich reported no fear reaction. When the EP practitioner tested this report by having Rich walk onto a nearby fire escape, he experienced no anxiety. Then, the practitioner asked Rich to recall several of his most intensive traumatic combat experiences, using the same tapping procedure. These experiences were "neutralized," to use an EP term, within an hour. Rich was given several homework assignments so that he could deal with other traumatic experiences as he recalled them. Within a few weeks, his insomnia cleared, and he stopped re-experiencing the combat memories. Within a few months, Rich discontinued his medication and checked himself out of the hospital. He never returned, and simply got on with his life— still practicing the EP rituals whenever he experienced stress. One case report does not validate an entire procedure, but Rich's story demonstrates how EP can be applied to PTSD.

EP is frequently combined with other treatments such as *Traumatic Incident Reduction,* a short-term treatment for PTSD. This approach operates on the principle that a resolution of the trauma is required, rather than a mere *catharsis* or discharge. Clients are encouraged to describe the traumatizing incident fully, in great detail, telling and retelling the practitioner everything that they remember about witnessing the murder at school, contributing to the battlefield killing of a child, or enduring a rape, a motor vehicle accident, an assault, bullying, harassment, or betrayal. Each retelling may evoke additional layers of thoughts, emotions, regrets, decisions, and opinions. These recapitulations may be accompanied by such EP procedures as tapping, or other adjuncts such as hypnosis, relaxation, or role-playing. In one study, positive results were obtained in less than two hours; like all such studies, of course, replications supervised by researchers with no connection to the approach are required before definite conclusions can be drawn (Stallard, 2006).

### Eye Movement Desensitization and Reprocessing (EMDR)

This unique process has obtained such positive results that U.S. government officials have placed it on their "approved" list for veterans' treatment. The *Eye Movement Desensitization and Reprocessing* (EMDR) approach asks the client to evoke visual images of a traumatic experience. At the same time, the client's attention is grounded on some type of stimulation such as a tapping sound, or— most frequently—back-and-forth eye movements as the client follows the practitioner's finger. This combination is felt to reduce the emotional charge associated with the traumatic experience, desensitizing the client. As the desensitization occurs, the practitioner guides the client through a process of restructuring and reframing in which the meaning of the distressing experience is transformed. For example, "I am always in danger" may become "I feel that I am safe."

Advocates of EMDR claim that talk therapies attempt to retrain the language centers of the brain to override the emotional centers, an often futile task. EMDR, on the other hand, is thought to work with the "whole brain," including the areas directly accessed by EMDR.

### Group Approaches

Not all psychotherapy or other interventions for PTSD are carried out on a one-to-one basis, group and family psychotherapies being the prime examples. A group can serve as a "safe haven" where clients feel comfortable sharing their feelings of isolation, resentments, interpersonal problems, flashbacks, and frightening nightmares. Dream-sharing groups have attained attention, thanks to the publicity given to them by the International Association for the Study of Dreams, which highlights PTSD nightmares in its journal, newsletter, and conferences.

One group facilitator encourages trauma survivors to interpret their own dreams and nightmares, opening up the discussion by having group members listen to a volunteer's dream report. Group members preface their contributions by saying, "If this were my dream, this is what it would mean to me." The dreamer accepts the insights with which he or she feels most comfortable, gradually arriving at an interpretation that can be put into practice the following days and weeks. This approach has been adapted for use on the Internet with positive results; in one study, participants disclosed more personal information those who were in similar face-to-face groups.

PTSD nightmares need little interpretation, as they usually are literal replays of the traumatic experience. A college student, Eufemio, had repeated nightmares about the night he was beaten within an inch of his life because of his sexual orientation. In this case, the group leader urged Eufemio to re-dream the nightmare immediately upon awakening, giving it a different ending. The group suggested a variety of endings: Eufemio could pull out a hidden gun and shoot his assailants. He could call police officers to the scene and have the perpetrators imprisoned. He could extend forgiveness to the gang, acknowledging their ignorance and stupidity. He could imagine that his strongest friends suddenly came out of the shadows to punish the malevolent assailants. Eufemio selected the latter option and practiced it diligently over the next few weeks. Much to his delight, the nightmares lessened in their intensity and their occurrence, finally disappearing entirely.

But the group leader pushed the resolution further, asking Eufemio what personal myth was revealed by his nightmare. Immediately, Eufemio stated, "I am always going to be at risk because I am gay." Group members suggested more positive personal myths that empowered Eufemio rather than exposed his weakness. Some of them were practical such as "I have learned not to walk back to the dormitories alone at night." Others were more philosophical, for example, "I am going to do so well at school that I will obtain respect even from people who dislike my sexual orientation." This volley of new personal myths had a "ripple effect" once Eufemio started to put them into practice. He found that he was sleeping better, making more friends, and his stress and anxiety level decreased, allowing him to excel in his coursework.

Sometimes group work can be effective without the presence of a psychotherapist. The dream group just described was led by a member of the International Association for the Study of Dreams, many of whose members do not have graduate degrees but have taken workshops and courses in "dreamwork." Some groups have no formal leader but allow people with similar backgrounds to discuss common issues, whether it is the aftermath of war combat, emotional harassment at work, or sexual abuse by trusted people such as relatives or athletic coaches. The well-known *twelve-step program* of Alcoholics Anonymous is also used by Gamblers Anonymous, Debtors Anonymous, Workaholics Anonymous, and groups where substance abuse, compulsive sex, or over-eating is a crucial issue. Advocates for family members and friends of addicted people organize support groups of *systems approaches* to behavior change.

When there is a psychotherapist present, his or her orientation provides the framework for the group. Psychodynamic, cognitive-behavioral, humanistic-existential, and mind-body groups are fairly common, and often focus on particular themes. For example, a group of PTSD survivors might deal with anger management, social skills training, relaxation or meditation, or other forms of psychoeducation. More specialized forms of group therapy include expressive psychotherapies such as those centered on art, dance, or music. Jacob L. Moreno's highly structured form of group therapy is known as *psychodrama* and cannot be employed outside of a group setting.

Following World War II, two British psychotherapists, S.H. Foulkes and Wilfred Bion, used group therapy to treat what was then known as "combat fatigue." A U.S. existential psychotherapist, Irvin Yalom, distilled the advantages of group therapy, citing the development of responsibility, trust, social skills, altruism, hope, and group cohesiveness, as well as the understanding of one's family background and what the group has in common. A 2005 study established the success of group psychotherapy in treating PTSD (Kanas, 2005).

Family psychotherapies date back to Alfred Adler. Since his pioneering efforts, they have taken many different forms, including Nathan Ackerman's psychodynamic approach, Virginia Satir's interest in family communication, and John Bowlby's (1988) emphasis on a child's original *attachments* to his or her caretakers. Family psychotherapists tend to see the family as a *system* and the PTSD survivor as representing a challenge to the equilibrium of that system.

*Couples counseling* highlights the relationship between the PTSD survivor and his or her spouse; it is not uncommon for a wife of a combat veteran to bemoan, "This is not the man I married; sometimes I think that his spirit is still in Iraq." A husband might share the statement "She is actually a different person since she returned from Afghanistan." The "significant other" of a rape survivor might observe a marked change in sexual intimacy. The partner of a person who survived an automobile crash might complain about the survivor's tendency to stay indoors most of the time. The fiancée of a robbery and assault survivor may observe a suspiciousness bordering on paranoia that dates back to the theft. All these comments are grist for the mill of a couples' counselor.

### Psychopharmacological Approaches

We have discussed how PTSD disrupts the balance between the hippocampus and the amygdala, on the one hand, and the prefrontal cortex, on the other. This network has failed to assimilate the traumatic memories, and PTSD has resulted from the destabilization, resulting in exaggerated anxiety, agitation, inhibition, dissociation, and flashbacks. *Psychopharmacotherapy*, the use of medication for therapeutic purposes, is an attempt to jumpstart the integration process, restoring some semblance of equilibrium to the brain and body. Furthermore, medication is less expensive than psychotherapy, so it is more timely and cost-effective. Some psychiatrists have abandoned the "psychotherapeutic hour" for 15-minute consultations, after which a prescription is given for an appropriate drug.

One psychiatrist, reporting her work at the Bronx Veterans' Administration Medical Center in New York, bragged that her therapy lasted for three months, followed by a "tune-up" in which her patients' medication could be adjusted. Many PTSD survivors view psychotherapy with suspicion, fearing it would leave a "stigma" on their military, school, or occupational record, which would be less likely if they were using prescribed drugs.

The major techniques in pharmacotherapy begin with selecting a drug whose actions might be expected to "normalize" the abnormalities associated with PTSD. At that point, monitoring and adjusting the dosage are provided to maximize therapeutic efficacy and minimize side effects. Finally, conclusions are drawn as to the drug's effectiveness for a particular client, based in part on his or her reports (Friedman, Davidson, & Stein, 2009).

You will notice that we put the word "normalize" in quotation marks; what is "normal" on the battlefield often is considered "abnormal" in civilian life. Healthy families often describe the "appropriate" behavior in an oppressive family as "inappropriate." Furthermore, many of the symptoms that categorize people as "disordered" are actually attempts to survive in a situation that is itself "disordered," namely, their survival in worlds not of their making. Practitioners who prescribe medication ignore these considerations; their prescriptions are basically well-meaning attempts to help the PTSD survivor "adjust," "cope," and "function." In this book, we have brought out readers' attention to the fact that many common terms as "social constructs" that may have little utility in another culture and that might have little validity in this culture when critically examined. A volley of books and research studies has questioned the long-term effectiveness of pharmacotherapy. In one of them, psychiatrist Daniel Carlat (2010) asks if psychiatry has sold its soul to the pharmaceutical industry. These caveats need to be kept in mind as we describe this field, which has spawned drugs that have become standard treatments for many PTSD survivors.

The most commonly used medications include *selective serotonin reuptake inhibitors* (SSRIs) and *serotonin and norepinephrine uptake inhibitors* (SNRIs). The former is a group of antidepressants, sold under such brand names as Paxil and Zoloft. The latter are a different class of antidepressants that are sold under such brand names as Prozac and Sarafem. *Monoamine oxidase inhibitors* (MAOIs) are used to combat re-experiencing trauma, while some anti-psychotic medications have been found to reduce social isolation, physical aggression, trauma-related hallucinations, and paranoia. For those who have negative reactions to the SSRIs and SNRIs, an older group of drugs, the *tricyclic antidepressants* (TCAs) can be used. Their brand names include Surmontil and Vivactil, but they were eclipsed in 1987 when Prozac hit the market and became the best-selling pharmaceutical product in history.

Considerable support for treating PTSD medically has been demonstrated by symptom relief. Several types of SSRIs, SNRIs, and TCAs have been effective in addressing such PTSD symptoms as inability to concentrate, anxiety, insomnia, depression, anger, explosive outbursts, hyperarousal, numbing, and flashbacks.

Certain *alpha-* and *beta-blockers*, such as Prazosin, have been used with great success in decreasing the incidence of nightmares (Peterson, et al., 2011). Long-term recurrence of trauma-related nightmares can severely impact one's overall functioning both during the day and at night. However, medications are not fully effective in treating nightmares or other PTSD symptoms if used in isolation. In fact, while medications will not provide successful recovery from trauma, they can allow for some stabilization of overwhelming symptoms, while psychotherapy and other interventions can address the invisible wounds of PTSD that conventional psychopharmacotherapy is ill-equipped to handle.

For this reason, we believe it is important to consider a radically different approach to psychopharmacotherapy, namely the use of *methylenedioxymeth-amphetamine* (MDMA) for PTSD. Better known as "Ecstasy," MDMA has short-term effects of six hours and long-term effects that depend upon the nature of the therapeutic alliance and follow-up. Like the SSRIs, it inhibits serotonin, but unlike the SSRIs, it need not be taken indefinitely. MDMA appears to increase activity in the prefrontal cortex, enhancing clients' sense of control and reducing their emotional avoidance. Because clients' cognitive skills do not appear to be affected by MDMA, new personal myths and beliefs can replace previous ones. Finally, with treatment by MDMA, they seem capable of discussing existential issues such as guilt, shame, and responsibility with their psychotherapist, a reaction rarely reported by users of the SSRIs or other more conventional medications.

In sum, there appears to be a legitimate role for psychopharmacotherapy in the treatment of PTSD, but it should be noted that the annals are filled with reports of unfavorable reactions, including suicides. Hence, the SSRIs and SNRIs are not magic bullets. There are even studies in which psychotherapy, especially CBT, performed as well as these medications. PTSD is a difficult condition to treat, and all approaches manifest failures that stand beside their successes.

## WHERE'S THE BEEF?

Psychopharmacotherapy can provide an in-depth understanding about the biological and neurological underpinnings of traumatic stress. Psychiatry has departed from Freud's psychodynamic legacy, becoming grounded in the neurobiochemical foundations of the individual. Although these psychiatric understandings are based on what is often referred to as the *biomedical model* of Western medicine, it has been useful in understanding and identifying symptoms.

Yet psychiatry's understanding of symptomology is limited. For example, it tends to categorize individuals' symptoms without considering that it is possible for people to experience PTSD symptomology without having undergone a traumatizing event. Paulson and Krippner (2009) have presented a spectrum of traumatic stress reactions, pointing out that such experiences as marital conflicts, employment difficulties, and chronic illness may activate symptomology related to an earlier trauma. Three out of four Americans claim that they are "stressed out" by something related to their job. Indeed, some describe work-related and marriage-related traumas as among the worst experience of their lives. These experiences, horrid as they may be, are sometimes assimilated without leaving long-lasting PTSD in their wake. The predisposing, activating, and maintaining causes and effects of PTSD are deeply enmeshed. Psychopharmacotherapy is linear in nature, while PTSD is usually non-linear. In other words, PTSD is too complex to yield readily to long-term resolution by medication alone.

Medications can be tested by administering a new drug to a group of PTSD survivors while giving a placebo, a substance that has no known medicinal effect, to a similar group. Even though a sizable number of the latter will improve, thanks to the *placebo effect*, if a large number of the former improve, the new drug is eventually approved. Psychotherapy research is not so easily accomplished. Placebo treatments can be used, such as talking with a bogus psychotherapist about the weather. Even so, many clients will improve simply because they are given attention.

Many physicians capitalize on their patients' response to *placebo medication*. A large number of people report fewer symptoms after they are given a sugar pill or other placebo, even though it has no active ingredients. The role of placebos cannot be overemphasized. They were an *adaptive trait* in human evolution, one that assisted the survival of the species.

### Evidence-based Treatments

In the United States, people who want to deliver psychotherapeutic services need to have a license from a program that has been approved by their state. And if they want to be reimbursed by the state for their services, they need to use an approach that is *evidence-based*, one that is backed up by a body of experimental work to support its usefulness.

Evaluating treatment approaches for PTSD is not a simple procedure. Do you remember the term "co-morbidity"? PTSD rarely occurs in isolation. It is usually combined with such other problems as drug addiction, depression, anxiety, and dissociation. Each of these conditions qualifies as a "disorder" according to the *Diagnostic and Statistical Manual of Mental Disorders*, or DSM. In addition, traumatic stress occurs on a spectrum; DSM calls it PTSD only if a number of symptoms are observed and experienced. Furthermore, PTSD can be *acute* or *chronic*, temporary or long-lasting. Sometimes a potentially traumatizing event such as a motor vehicle accident will evoke one or two sleepless nights, with no sequels. At other times, PTSD kicks in a few weeks or even a few months after the traumatizing event takes place. In addition, there are predisposing factors that may themselves deserve a DSM diagnosis.

Keeping all these issues in mind, a 2008 study evaluated several *bona fide treatments* for PTSD. By *bona fide*, the authors meant mainstream psychotherapies for which enough research had been conducted for comparisons to be made. The approaches were evaluated in terms of guidelines created by the International Society for Traumatic Stress Studies, similar to guidelines used by the American Psychiatric Association, the Veterans Administration, the U.S. Department of Defense, and similar groups in Great Britain and Australia. The approaches in this study receiving an "A" rating were prolonged exposure therapy, cognitive processing therapy, stress-inoculation therapy (a form of CBT), EMDR, and certain types of medication (Benish et al., 2008). And the other bona fide approaches were not far behind.

Several similar studies went a bit further and identified the common elements among effective psychotherapies. They were summarized in a 2010 article concluding that the most effective of the treatments focused on clients' memories of their traumatic experiences and the meanings they had for them. These trauma-focused psychotherapies fared better than less directive, unstructured interventions. Some approaches, such as transpersonal and humanistic-existential psychotherapies, clinical hypnosis, mind-body approaches, and REBT, could not be properly evaluated because the research literature contained an inadequate number of long-term investigations.

In response to the 2008 study's suggestion that all bona fide treatments were effective, the 2010 study agreed that this was the case. Nevertheless, some treatments are more effective than others (Ehlers et al., 2010). One result that surprised many people was the finding that medication without psychotherapy seemed to be not as effective as psychotherapy without medication (Krystal et al., 2011).

### Do Not Forget the Psychotherapist

The therapeutic alliance has been discussed since the advent of formal psychotherapy, but in 2011, Charles Gelso revised the concept and identified its two major components. The first is *genuineness*, the intent to avoid deception, and the second is *realism*, perceiving and experiencing the other person in ways that benefit the client. These two components are more important than transference, unconscious projections, or any of the other dimensions conjectured by the early psychoanalysts.

This finding is especially important in the case of PTSD survivors, less than half of whom receive treatment. And of this number, another half drop out after one or two sessions. The reason most frequently cited is that they could not form a satisfactory relationship with the practitioner. In other words, all major psychotherapies appear to be effective, but the same thing cannot be said for the psychotherapists themselves.

## Conclusion

Psychotherapeutic treatment of PTSD has a significant, if not crucial, impact on many clients' recovery from trauma. In addition, psychotherapy that is implemented in conjunction with medication increases the possibility of such recovery. There are many psychotherapeutic approaches that can address the symptoms of PTSD and each one involves some way of listening to the client's story. Simply repeating the events that led to a traumatic experience is not quite enough; psychotherapeutic treatment will not succeed unless it translates that story into a changed personal myth and revamped patterns of behavior. For example, when dealing with nightmares, the client may create an alternative ending or scenario to the nightmare and replay it in his or her mind. Eventually, this replay will alter the content of the nightmare itself. Once the nightmare changes, other symptoms may fall like dominos because a deep part of the client's psyche has been accessed and transformed.

As researchers have suggested, approaching clients holistically and individualizing their treatment can facilitate working with the unique symptoms and needs of each of them. For example, a psychotherapist could develop a humanistic-existential foundation for conceptualizing the nature of trauma and then incorporate techniques, as needed, from CBT, mindfulness meditation, the expressive arts, or other approaches in addressing PTSD and its symptoms.

Future forms of treatment need to address the issue of suicide among people with PTSD diagnoses. They need to incorporate friends, family members, and support groups in the treatment program. They need to find ways to treat or "debrief" people quickly, once the traumatizing event has occurred; and to use the Internet and other technologies to deliver services to those traumatized people who want help but are not getting it. Each of these initiatives will empower PTSD clients, helping them to trust themselves and others, and to work through the wounds their trauma has afflicted upon their souls.

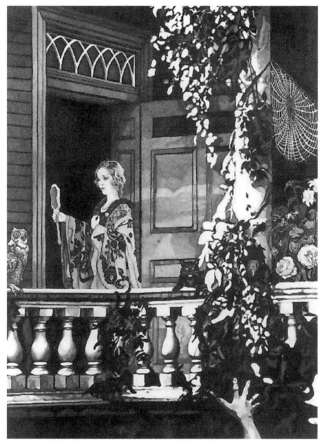

Piazza Piece (Reproduced from the original art of Dierdre Luzwick.)

# 8

# The Positive Side of PTSD: Post-traumatic Strengths

As we enter our discussion of "post-traumatic strengths," it may be help-ful to remember that optimal mental health is not a static state. It is not a condition that we eventually reach and that remains perpetual and unchanging. The inner climate of our experience can be likened to the outer climate of weather patterns—it is often unpredictable and always changing. The ebb and flow of mental health and well-being in this sense are dynamic; they move in tandem with the rhythms of our life experiences. Periods of strength and vitality, or conversely times of stress and fragility, can be seen as natural expressions of the totality of the human experience. Though PTSD is not some-thing we would wish upon anyone, there is, nevertheless, "gold to mine" within its spectrum.

People seek to avoid pain and suffering, yet paradoxically their greatest challenges often help them discover what is most meaningful in their lives. In meeting the range of complex struggles that PTSD survivors experience, strengths can emerge that may otherwise have remained outside of awareness. Combat veterans sometimes can recall instances of courage and leadership that were overlooked during their times of anguish. For example, women and men who were raped can utilize the strategies that kept the sexual assault from turning into a murder. Survivors of motor vehicle accidents can draw upon instant life or death decisions that may have saved their lives.

Trauma sometimes leads to long-lasting personality change. Several forms of suffering incurred through traumatic experiences can bypass a person's defenses, thereby opening the pathway to greater compassion and awakening receptivity to the suffering and injustices in the world. It is precisely this receptivity that can lead PTSD survivors toward a life of deeper connection and meaning. Survivors of genocides, terrorist attacks, and torture chambers often give inspirational lectures to audiences of all ages, making no secret of the ongoing residues of their ordeals in the form of PTSD symptoms.

Growth after a traumatic experience can involve a shift from conventional, conditioned behaviors to those that reflect more authentic choices. Conventional behavior, such as going to school, having a job, wending one's way through relationships, and behaving in a predictable way all reflect abodes where most people reside. The values that most people hold emerge through conventional norms and the prevailing cultural myths. In the case of PTSD, however, the circumstances that gave rise to it—for example, experiencing war, assaults, or an aircraft collision—can shake the values that had previously informed one's life. These values no longer fit or made sense after experiencing trauma that fell outside of an individual's expectations of normality, fairness, and justice.

This challenge offers an opportunity to look beyond conventional ways of living and find values, personal myths, and worldviews that more appropriately fit one's experiences. In some cases, people may remain stuck at a level where they survive but do not really flourish. Others, however, transform their post-traumatic stress through engaging in a journey toward positive growth. Throughout this book, we have discussed the case of Daryl Paulson whose descent into alcoholism followed his combat-induced PTSD, but he pulled himself together, attended graduate school, and became a successful executive and author (Paulson, 1994).

In another example of personal transformation, we present the case of Howard Wasdin, a member of the U.S. Navy's elite Sea, Air, and Land (SEAL) team, who survived combat in Mogadishu, Ethiopia. He terminated his tour of duty with three bullets in his leg, forcing his retirement, and leaving him with chronic pain and PTSD. He thought that having PTSD was a weakness, but his wife urged him to write about his experiences, saying this would be great therapy for him. At first he dismissed this idea, but his wife kept insisting that he get started. Finally, he and Stephan Temple (2011) wrote *SEAL Team 6: Memoirs of an Elite Naval SEAL Sniper* and his symptoms began to disappear. He recalled the physical training he received and the quick decisions he had to make. He began to visit a firing range and discovered that he enjoyed target shooting, even though it was now for recreation. His muscles remembered the training he had received, despite his wounds. Telling one's story has been a useful means of recovering from trauma over the millennia (Mehl-Madrona, 2010). Needless to say, it is not a panacea, and there must be a suitable time, place, and audience, so that this disclosure does not re-traumatize the narrator.

In another case, Rina, a high school teacher, was a child in Angola during the civil war that devastated her native country for decades. She still cringes when she hears a helicopter overhead, even though she now lives in Switzerland where these vehicles serve civilian purposes. However, telling her stories of surviving years under life-threatening conditions to her classes provides her an emotional relief, as well as utilizing the trauma in a positive way. Aside from her reaction to helicopters, the symptoms of traumatic stress have not returned. Nonetheless, it took Rina several years before she could share her experiences. She took the advice of a naïve friend to talk about her experiences as soon as she left the country. But each time she tried to do this, she broke down in tears and flashed back to the war zone. Sensibly, Rina waited until she could relate her experiences with composure and without having an adverse reaction.

The leap in growth that is possible following an exposure to trauma versus returning to one's familiar baseline functioning (or even regressing to a lower level of performance) has led to an area of research known as "post-traumatic growth." This term, coined by Richard Tedeschi and Richard Calhoun (1996), refers to positive personal changes that can result from the struggle to deal with trauma and its psychological consequences. In the complex aftermath of a traumatizing event, individuals struggle in their efforts toward recovery. As previously noted, while engaged in this struggle, trauma survivors are often forced to re-evaluate previously held worldviews. Post-traumatic growth occurs when individuals are able to formulate more adaptive interpretations or worldviews following a terrible event that traumatizes them. This personal growth can be measured by adaptations in perceived changes in self-concept, relationships with others, philosophy of life, spirituality, and other new possibilities (Schultz, Tallman, & Altmaier, 2010; Tedeschi & McNally, 2011).

It is important to note that, although the formal framing of post-traumatic growth occurred fairly recently, the recognition that suffering and tragedy can elicit personal transformation is longstanding. The general realization that suffering and distress can potentially yield positive change is thousands of years old. Religions and philosophies such as Christianity, Judaism, Hinduism, Buddhism, Islam, and Confucianism as well as shamanic tales, Nordic epics, Native American legends, Greek classics, and other narratives, have long portrayed circumstances in which personal adversity is the catalyst for developing a deeper relationship to one's soul, the most fundamental part of one's psyche. Attempts to understand and discover the meaning of suffering appear in the works of novelists, dramatists, and poets, and have been a central theme in philosophical inquiry.

The *testimony method* is a psychological intervention that originated as a means of treating survivors of the Nazi Holocaust, political violence, and torture. In Chile, this method is referred to as a *testimonio*, introduced in the 1970s as a way to combat post-traumatic experiences related to political oppression. Clients are encouraged to narrate their traumatic experiences. Telling one's story allows clients to redefine their experiences and attach new and different meanings to them. These stories can be told to a therapist, a group of fellow survivors, or to a close acquaintance. It permits the traumatic experience to be externalized and integrated in a new way, especially if the audience is accepting and demonstrates empathy. Women, in particular, seem to benefit from this approach since it validates personal experiences that may have been belittled by men in positions of authority who often downgrade the severity of the trauma (McKinney, 2007).

Carl Rogers felt that traumatized individuals have vast personal resources for self-understanding and that these can be tapped if several conditions are met. The psychotherapist, acquaintance, or group needs to take a genuine interest in the person telling the story, demonstrating a high degree of empathy and an unconditional acceptance of the trauma survivor. But timing is also important; in some instances (with combat being one of them) an immediate intervention is appropriate, but in other instances (witnessing an act of violence) a period of time needs to elapse before the narration can be therapeutic. Most New Yorkers who immediately gave counselors their reactions to witnessing the 9/11 terrorist attacks did not appear to benefit from this intervention.

"What doesn't kill you makes you stronger" is one of the best-known statements of Friedrich Nietzsche, the German philosopher. Nietzsche was a founder of existential philosophy, the investigation into how people can bring meaning into their lives, even to traumatizing events. Nietzsche also wrote that "to live is to suffer; to survive is to find some meaning in the suffering." Existential psychotherapists believe that their approach is especially pertinent to dealing with PTSD.

In 2011, the U.S. Department of Defense admitted that the rate of combat veteran suicides was still high, averaging one per day, despite the millions of dollars that had been spent on preventive and remedial programs. We would suggest that better results might be obtained from counseling and psychotherapeutic approaches that attempt to penetrate the very core of one's life world, focusing on what makes sense, what does not make sense, and what one can do about it. Nothing need escape scrutiny. There should be no "sacred cows." If one's religious beliefs, patriotic ideals, family traditions, ethnic heritage, medications (legal or illegal), and personal relationships have not provided support to a fragile psyche, they need to be revamped or jettisoned. In every sense of the word, this is a life and death matter. Discarding a useless personal myth or unsatisfactory relationship is the easy step; finding a replacement is the arduous part of the journey. There are many potential companions, psychotherapies, faiths (including the lack of faith), and insights available in the Internet, in self-help groups, in neighborhood resource centers, and even in bars and athletic centers that may yield surprises. Seek and ye shall find!

## EVIDENCE AND CHARACTERISTICS
## OF POST-TRAUMATIC GROWTH

A key feature of post-traumatic stress is that it can lead to a post-traumatic strength by increasing resiliency to future adversity. Some research studies suggest that post-traumatic growth is far more common than long-term post-traumatic stress disorder. This body of research indicates that most human beings naturally adapt and grow following trauma (Fretwell & Baldwin-Kiland, 2011). This makes sense from the perspective of human evolution; if traumatized men and women could not recover from human-made conflict and from natural disasters such as earthquakes, they would not live long enough to have descendants. If they were resilient, however, their genes would be passed on to future generations.

An example of this can be seen in the case of former U.S. prisoners of war (POWs) who spent up to eight years in North Vietnam's infamous "Hanoi Hilton" prison. Research studies determined that most of the former prisoners experienced positive growth after the experience, along with a PTSD rate of only 4 percent. In fact, those who experienced the worst trauma, which included repeated torture, starvation, solitary confinement, and physical abuse over many years, reported the most personal growth in the decades following their release. One critical factor was the camaraderie of the prisoners; POWs supported each other, with the strongest of the group serving as role models to those who might have fallen apart without their example. While none of the POWs expressed a desire to go through the experience again, a number of them reported that they were now sturdier and tougher because of it. In addition, a great deal of research has shown that post-traumatic growth is related to greater levels of positive well-being, acceptance, and optimistic ways of dealing with future stress.

Another research study, which utilized data from the National Vietnam Readjustment Study, found that 70 percent of male veterans regarded their military experience as mainly positive. According to the researchers, there was no convincing evidence that these positive reflections conveyed what psychotherapists call "pathological defensive denial," the tendency to cover up something negative by making a positive statement. The interpretation of the data was viewed as consistent with successful adaptation to war zone experiences and what followed (Tedeschi & McNally, 2011). Once again, it is not the event that is crucial; it is the way that one interprets the event that can lead to strength or to weakness, to growth or to frailty.

Former U.S. POWs have contributed a great deal to psychologists' understanding of post-traumatic growth. Based on the Post-traumatic Growth Inventory (PTGI), 30 aviators who had been POWs of the North Vietnamese were assessed (Feder et al., 2008). Nearly two-thirds of the men expressed at least moderate post-traumatic growth, and slightly over one-third reported a great or very great degree of growth. Such PTGI categories as Personal Strength and Appreciation for Life showed the most prominent effect. In addition, post-traumatic growth remained consistent among the former POWs whether or not PTSD was present. Moreover, such traits as optimism were positively related to post-traumatic growth. And the longer a POW was a captive, the more post-traumatic growth was indicated (Tedeschi & McNally, 2011). The life of John McCain, who was imprisoned in North Vietnamese POW camps for many years, is a prime example of post-traumatic growth, as he went on to become a U.S. Senator and presidential candidate.

Some cultures also manifest this point of view. Post-traumatic strengths can be seen in Japan's capacity to rebuild itself into one of the world's greatest intellectual, economic, and industrial powers following World War II, during which some three Japanese million deaths are estimated to have occurred. And again, after the 2011 earthquake, tsunami devastation, and nuclear emergency in Japan, Prime Minister Kan reminded the Japanese of their history of resiliency, strength, and determination to overcome adversity. Such an invocation is a key factor in resiliency itself. The Japanese held the perspective that they had the vigor, knowledge, and stamina to survive, because their nation had already lived through other adversities.

Haiti may be the poorest country in the Western hemisphere. but it boasts the largest percentage of professional artists. Within weeks of the 2010 earthquake that devastated the capital, Port-au-Prince and much of the countryside, Haiti's painters and sculptors were completing new works of art to replace the thousands of museum and gallery pieces that had been destroyed. The same can be said of individual trauma survivors; the determination and insight that can emerge through surviving a trauma may become a new capability for strength propelling a confidence in one's capacity to survive future adversity. As the Spanish philosopher George Santayana once wrote, "The truth is cruel, but it can be loved, and it makes free those who have loved it."

An important point to note is that post-traumatic growth and resiliency are not quite the same. For example, highly resilient people may experience less post-traumatic growth than less resilient people. The reason for this is easy to understand. Resilient men and women already have strong coping skills and are less likely to struggle with the psychological effects of trauma; thus, they do not experience a new range of opportunities to grow and to change. Resiliency indicates one's capacity to "bounce back" from an adverse experience. But the "bounce" is less noticeable among those who are already resilient than among those who have to fight hard to recover.

Gender differences also have been explored. Research consistently shows females reporting higher levels of both PTSD and post-traumatic growth than males (Tedeschi & Calhoun, 1996). However, little is known about these differences. One suggestion is that females tend to use positive religious coping skills more frequently than do men. Since faith can be a powerful factor in surviving trauma, this difference may partially explain why females report higher levels of post-traumatic growth since positive religious coping is related to post-traumatic growth, and a lack of religious coping is related to more PTSD symptoms. These relationships continue to be significant even after researchers make sure that other types of coping styles such as focusing on the problem, focusing on emotion, and avoidance do not account for the difference.

Many psychotherapists explore their clients' faith or lack of faith. A trauma survivor need not be a member of an organized religion to have faith. Being "spiritual" can be just as helpful as being "religious." And there are many atheists and agnostics who have a positive philosophy of life that sustains them in times of adversity. Of course, some people are both spiritual and religious. It is those who are not spiritual, positive, or religious who seem to lack meaning in their lives, and who are at risk for a slow recovery from PTSD and its symptoms.

Hidalgo, a young man from New Mexico, stopped going to Mass because the Roman Catholic priest told the congregation that gay men and lesbian women were doomed to spend eternity in Hell. However, Hidalgo considered himself to be spiritual, treating people with kindness and respect, enjoying time spent in nature, taking nursing courses in college, and devoting himself to his boyfriend with a single-minded passion. However, Hidalgo was in for a rude surprise. He shared his story with us.

> The most traumatic experience in my life was breaking up with my boyfriend Rodrigo. Even though we had broken up many times over the years, I knew we would always get back together again no matter how badly the incident had ended. We met through social networking. I had never met a boyfriend through Facebook before but there was something about him that attracted me. When we finally met face to face three years ago, it seemed like instant love. Rodrigo made me so damn happy and feel so damn special. I had never felt this way about anyone before. We had something going that I had never experienced before in my life.

But two years into the relationship I found out Rodrigo was cheating on me. I confronted him with this and he denied it. Frankly, I wouldn't have minded it so much if he just would have been honest with me. But after this confrontation, he started to beat me. I am a peaceful guy and would never think of inflicting pain on someone I loved. It was the beatings rather than the cheating that led me to break up with him. One night we had been at a party, and he had passed out on the rug when we came back to our apartment. I stared at him, and saw him with his head lying in his own vomit on a dirty carpet, and I realized he would never change. I just got up, phoned my sister to pick me up, and left. I took as much of my stuff as I could carry, wrote him a letter, and walked out the door.

When I got to my sister's house I felt that my life was over. I really had no reason to live. I wanted to die right there, knowing that I would not be sleeping with him that night. I loved him so much. I went into deep depression. I had suicidal thoughts. I suffered from depression and anxiety all through the day and for the next several months. Rodrigo wanted me to come back, but I resolved to be strong. No more beatings, no more lies, no more ridicule. I could never put up with that again. He told me, "You left me because you don't love me, and you have found someone else." This was not true. But he refused to take any responsibility himself. I told him, "I did not stop loving you or because I loved someone else. I left because I started loving myself."

My church did not help me one damn bit with this process. In fact, the priests kept telling me that I was committing sinful acts. I had a support group consisting of friends who were both gay and straight. And I was able to find the "God within," as one of my friends put it. It took a while, but now the suicidal thoughts are gone. Little by little, my anxiety and depression have decreased. The stronger I became, the better I started to feel. For the first time in my life, I really love myself.

When I was a teenager, I was teased and beaten up because I was gay. I carried around this self-hatred for too many years. I got the love I needed from my boyfriends, especially Rodrigo. But now I know I am strong enough to keep from even considering going back to Rodrigo. And I am getting the love I need from my "Higher Self," to use another term a friend gave me. I am in no rush to find another boyfriend. I am enjoying my own company, and am anything but lonely. In fact, I feel beloved and blessed.

## MODELS OF POST-TRAUMATIC GROWTH

When used by PTSD researchers and psychotherapists, a "model" is a concise description of a complicated phenomenon. One model of post-traumatic growth was developed by Ronnie Janoff-Bulman (1992). This model proposes that emotion and thought processes help the survivor rebuild a new worldview after trauma shatters his or her earlier assumptions about the world and the way it works. This model identifies three kinds of post-traumatic growth processes: (1) strength through suffering, (2) strength through existential re-evaluation, and (3) strength through psychological preparedness. A survivor can grow by working through the pain of the trauma, finding new ways of making life meaningful, being prepared to avoid future traumas, or by all three.

Tedeschi and Calhoun (1996) expanded upon these processes to create an evolving model of post-traumatic growth. The resulting model describes how several factors have the ability to increase the possibility of psychological growth following trauma. These include:

- the survivor's ability to think through the trauma and confront the issues it brings up;
- the survivor's ability to disclose one's concerns surrounding traumatic experiences and observe other peoples' reactions to this self-disclosure;
- the social and cultural contexts in which the trauma took place as well as the survivor's attempts to process, disclose, and resolve the trauma;
- the personal dispositions of the survivor and the degree to which he or she is resilient; and
- the degree to which specific traumatic experiences foster or suppress these processes.

There are also models for implementing the prevention of PTSD. Interventions have been developed as a means to foster resilience before the stressors occur in the hope that they will offset the occurrence of PTSD. An example of this can be seen in the U.S. Army's Comprehensive Soldier Fitness program. This training aims to increase a soldier's psychological and emotional fitness prior to deployment. The assumption underlying this approach is that this type of training will provide a foundation for post-traumatic growth following a soldier's exposure to those stressors that have the potential to become traumatizing events. It is rooted in positive psychology and uses a survey that attempts to measure soldiers' resilience in five core areas: (1) physical status, (2) emotional status, (3) family status, (4) social relationships, and (5) spirituality. If a soldier's responses fall into a "red area" in one or more of these areas, he or she is required to participate in a classroom or online course to strengthen their resilience.

As of mid-2011, close to one million U.S. soldiers had taken this survey; the results of this program are yet to be seen. Throughout the process, however, the model proposes that those who go to fight a war will absorb a lifesaving message. The message is that PTSD is not the inevitable outcome of combat, and if it is present, there are other aspects of post-traumatic living that can be mined for great value. With an early understanding of this possibility, soldiers may be in a better position to receive help after their deployment. And this assistance needs to emphasize the positive growth opportunities that are possible for them.

But the U.S. Army's Comprehensive Soldier Fitness program is not without its critics. One alleged flaw involves the spiritual area, which critics claim is too heavily weighted toward orthodox "believers" and discriminates against "free-thinkers." Defenders of the program insist that the spiritual area is not related to religiosity, but measures a person's core values and beliefs regarding their meaning and purpose in life. However, critics respond that the survey questions, as currently stated, are unconstitutional, claiming that they violate the separation of church and state.

Another criticism is that the program takes a simplistic approach to avoiding PTSD, attempting to substitute positive thoughts for unhappy and negative ones. In so doing, the program overlooks existential issues such as guilt, shame, and the questioning of the U.S. Army's mission in such parts of the world as Afghanistan, the site of U.S.'s longest-lasting war. Is this program inoculation or indoctrination? Time will tell, but critics maintain that soldiers deserve to be treated with greater respect rather than as participants in a massive social experiment (Leopold, 2011).

## THE JOURNEY HOME: CONDITIONS
## FOR POST-TRAUMATIC GROWTH

The "journey home" for PTSD survivors needs to help them construct positive meaning out of their hardships. This path is unique to each person and will take different forms. As discussed in previous chapters, psychotherapeutic approaches such as cognitive-behavioral and humanistic-existential psychotherapies are one such form, and an important one. Especially crucial is the search to discover positive meanings in a traumatic experience, during which time the significance of one's life can be evaluated. A great deal has been written about this process in the humanistic-existential work of such psychotherapists as Victor Frankl, James Bugental, and Rollo May. These writers have described how issues of choice, freedom, responsibility, meaning, tragedy, loneliness, and alienation can serve as rich resources for reconstructing a new personal mythology. The process itself—of questioning the meaning of one's existence—offers the possibility of authentically coming to terms with life. However, before the deepest layers of meaning are made visible, there is usually a period of turmoil and tension that must be lived through and endured.

Spiritual traditions, ranging from shamanism to Buddhism to Christian mysticism, have referred to this profoundly challenging period as the "dark night of the soul." This metaphor, attributed to the 16th-century Spanish mystic, St. John of the Cross, describes the spiritual crisis that occurs in the journey of the soul. Ultimately, the soul attains a level of detachment from its physical home in order to reach "the light," the union with God, or contact with the Great Spirit. Some Buddhist texts use the term "insight toward awakening," an appropriate description of this process. When one is experiencing the dark night of the soul, all previous existing forms of relief fall away, and one must find the inner strength to exist in the chaos. Eventually, if one works long and hard enough, order emerges from this chaos and darkness yields to light as the suffering is transcended.

In the case of trauma survivors, they may feel abandoned because their previous personal myths and beliefs no longer match the reality of their experience. This can result in what many tribal shamans term as "soul loss." Helping individuals with soul loss is a major shamanic function, and many of the descriptions of soul loss parallel those of PTSD. Fawn Journeyhawk, a Native American shaman, claims to take a shamanic journey back to her client's traumatizing event, recovering the lost soul, and bringing it into her client's physical body. This is followed by a regimen of contemplation, cleansing rituals, and lifestyle changes to anchor the soul so that it does not wander away. These new behaviors could include confronting such feelings as isolation and suspiciousness, as well as improving one's relationships and work performance.

But as difficult as this breakdown may be, the dark night is regarded by mystics, shamans, and others as a blessing in disguise. As the psychiatrist R.D. Laing observed:

> True sanity entails in one way or another the dissolution of the normal ego, that false self competently adjusted to our alienated social reality: the emergence of the inner archetypal mediators of divine power, and through this death a rebirth, and the eventual re-establishment of a new servant of the divine, no longer its betrayer. (Laing, 1983, p. 144)

In this sense, the disintegration that can occur through the experience and aftermath of trauma sets the stage for an abandonment of harmful cultural and personal myths and a subsequent rebirth into one's own authentic existence.

The path toward this growth can be further approached from an investigation of one's life journey. It would also take into account of the apparent inherent violation from the trauma, and the need to face the continuing effects of its aftermath. These aftereffects typically include the extended loneliness, the discouragement of putting one's job and career on hold, the feeling of being betrayed by spouses and lovers, and the loss of innocence—the realization that righteousness, fairness, and benevolence are often in short supply. All of these aftereffects reflect the erosion of belief in a just world, one of the most frequent personal myths that can be challenged by the trauma.

In the investigation of a larger perspective that extends beyond the immediate or remembered experience, the individual with PTSD can discover what the ancient Greeks called the *telos*, or end goal. This *telos* places the trauma within a larger field of meaning as the survivor creates a new personal mythology.

Clearly, the assistance of a psychotherapist, teacher, or spiritual guide is invaluable in this process. Without this assistance, recovery and strength-building may not be achieved, leaving those with PTSD marooned in the "there and then," rather than in the "here and now." They may become trapped in a life dictated entirely by the past rather than one in which is there is joy in the present and hope for the future. With assistance, individuals are better equipped to discover personal values that are transformed by their experiences.

However, many PTSD survivors discover these values without the help of a professional practitioner. By appealing to a "higher power" or by relying on their own common sense, they may become aware of the distinct post-traumatic strengths that belong to them. They can recover from within, adopting the character traits or powerful personal attributes that are uniquely their own, integrating them into their present lives.

This newfound strength could take the form of resilience, compassion, courage, or any number of what positive psychologists call "virtues." Whatever it might be, this is the reward that has been earned, the completion of their journey. This prize may be honored by a small support group or by a large community. Nonetheless, it marks the end of one's arduous voyage and the beginning of a new one.

### Hector's Story

An example of the strength that may be developed after PTSD can be seen in the case of Hector Aristizabal. Hector grew up in the barrios of Medellín, Colombia, where he and his siblings had to use all their wit, craftiness, and resources to endure poverty, the ever-present allure of cheap drugs and dangerous money, and the endemic violence from left-wing guerrillas, right-wing death squads, cocaine cartels, and the armed power of the police and the army.

In 1982, when Hector was 22 years old, Colombia's political climate was such that the president had urged his fellow patriots to "protect and defend the country" by reporting suspected subversive or terrorist activity. Colombia's "Patriot Act"—the *Estatuto de Seguridad*—allowed the government to arrest without a warrant or subsequent trial those suspected of being terrorists or having terrorist sympathies. At the time, Hector was a young actor and psychology student, privileged to be one of the rare few accepted into the University of Antioquia program in psychoanalysis. He combined his studies with theatrical work, having long been interested in the arts.

Hector was at home studying when soldiers came knocking on the door. After his mother answered and let them in, they began to raid the house in search of "subversive material." A horrified Hector watched as they reached under a mattress and pulled out a Marxist pamphlet. Despite his best efforts to keep the place clean of anything suspicious, his heart sank as he recognized the pamphlet that had belonged to his brother, Fernando. Later, he discovered that it had been a priest who had reported Fernando. During a camping trip with friends, the priest had offered several young people shelter from the rain and had overheard them talking about politics.

Hector and his brother were both seized by the military and held at Batallon Bombona, a military headquarter (though when his family inquired into their sons whereabouts, this was denied). After arriving, Hector was blindfolded and placed against a wall, his back toward a line of soldiers. As gunshots were fired, he was terrified, certain his end was near. Then to his surprise, he found himself still alive. It had been a mock execution. The soldiers then threw him into a dark prison cell and began to beat him repeatedly. After days deprived of water, he finally asked for a drink. His drink arrived in the form of having his head thrust repeatedly underwater to the verge of drowning—a torture technique called "waterboarding." Later they hung Hector from a pole, his body stretched like an animal. In a scene reminiscent of the now infamous Abu Ghraib prison pictures, they then administered electric shock to his genitals. After ten days of torture, Hector was finally released. He later left the country and moved to the United States.

Hector struggled for many years with the rage he felt and his desire to inflict violence on those responsible for his trauma. He even went so far as to make fun of his friends in the peace movement, saying that "there could be no peace without justice." In 1999, another tragedy occurred, when Hector's brother Fernando was abducted by a right-wing paramilitary group. Hector immediately returned to Colombia to help search for him. On the day of his arrival, his brother's body was found in a ditch beside the highway. Hector chose to be an observer at the autopsy, where he witnessed the effects of the unimaginable atrocities that had been committed while his brother had been held captive before he was killed. Again, Hector's feelings of rage were rekindled, so much so that he found himself planning a suicidal mission to kill those responsible.

Hector survived his ordeal through finding meaning in it, which he did through channeling his desire for revenge into constructive social action. After earning a master's degree in marriage and family therapy, he went on to combine his training in psychology and the arts with the lessons he had gained from his life experiences. He began working with other trauma survivors who had been tortured, incarcerated youth, immigrant families, and people affected by AIDS. He also uses theatrical performances as part of the movement to end torture and to challenge the U.S.'s alleged support of torture in many parts of Latin America. This led to the creation of "ImaginAction," an organization that offers programs all around the world to help people tap the transformative power of theatre for community building and reconciliation, strategizing, and individual healing and liberation.

"Any time you go through a difficult ordeal," Hector stated, "it can awaken inner resources and reveal strengths. In my own life," he went on to share, "I prefer to see post-traumatic stress as an essential part of the healing process rather than pathological symptoms that need eradication." Though symptoms of PTSD such as nightmares and intrusive thoughts are not foreign to him, he describes them as "the psyche calling attention to the wound as it seeks to rebuild itself."

> To remember, to put the pieces back together. I ask myself what my psyche is trying to say. What needs to be forgiven and absolved? What do I need to understand and learn? I don't resist revisiting the wound, but fight against obsessive thoughts of my weakness. Instead, I go back to find out what made me strong enough to survive. (Aristizabal & Lefer, 2010, p. 101)

Though Hector is quick to say that he does not claim the title of a shaman, he considers his journey to have been a shamanistic experience. He observed:

> The shaman is someone who has undergone a break with the reality most of us rely on. His or her identity has disintegrated. He or she has descended into hell, but also has returned, and that means he or she knows the path. He or she can go and come back, descend and return, and from those terrible depths the shaman brings back medicine and knowledge.
>
> Since my arrest and torture, I have carried the knowledge of how fragile we are, how tenuous our safety. I know I can fall apart again and have done so. But, I've also had the experience of rebuilding myself, and that too I know I can do. The shaman doesn't merely return from hell for his own sake. So I feel I must bring healing to those who've been to hell and are finding it hard to rediscover the path back to life on their own. Initiation remains at the stage of ordeal unless I find a way to share the gift of medicine I found with my wound. (Aristizabal & Lefer, 2010, p. 104)

Shamans were the first practitioners who performed rituals similar to the sessions led by today's psychotherapists and spiritual counselors. So it is appropriate to remember that what is today labeled PTSD is as old as humanity itself.

Glen Kulik who was repeatedly sexually abused at the age of 10 by a friend's uncle exemplifies these survival skills. He told nobody about the abuse, degenerated into homelessness, alcoholism, and drug addiction to dull the pain and shame. He failed to help a friend who was a fellow victim, and so guilt was added to the list of emotional reactions. While at the "bottom of the barrel," he found a psychotherapist willing to help him. He recovered, got married, became a father, and went on to found a facility for sober living in Los Angeles.

The term "bottom of the barrel" goes back to Roman times when it described the sediment left at the bottom of a wine barrel after the beverage is siphoned off. Cicero referred to the dregs of Roman society as the "bottom of the barrel" and Alcoholics Anonymous often uses to term to describe alcoholics who can only start their recovery after they have "bottomed out." The term certainly applies to Kulik as well as to Allen Martin, a California sheriff's deputy who was abused by a Roman Catholic priest for several years, starting when he was eight. His father refused to believe him, and he decided it was useless to tell anyone else. As a young adult, he "hit bottom" but was able to pull his life together. Those two stories are part of a remarkable film, *Boyhood Shadows: I Vowed I'd Never Tell*, developed by filmmakers Terri DeBono and Steve Rosen. They had created a 30-second public service announcement to publicize the services of a rape crisis center for male abuse survivors. They were astonished at the number of referrals that resulted, and decided to make a film about the topic. The group featured in their documentary is one of some 40 similar groups in the United States.

The reaction to the public service announcement underscores the importance of bringing the topic of PTSD to public awareness. A Florida psychotherapist, Carlos Zalaquett, worked with a 64-year-old client who had been referred to him for depression. She complained of experiencing depression and anxiety for the last four years so her family attributed her condition to "old age." However, when she mentioned to Zalaquett that she would like to drive her automobile again, the astute psychotherapist probed further. He discovered that his client had survived a near-death car accident four years previously and realized that she was a PTSD survivor. Using systematic desensitization, mental imagery, and actual exposure to driving, Zalaquett was able to turn around her condition within four months. Her anxiety and depression ceased and she developed a new post-traumatic strength—driving friends to psychotherapy in her own automobile.

Saleh Bien of Indonesia has provided a first-person account of what it is like to survive a motor vehicle accident only to fall prey to PTSD with its harrowing symptoms.

I remember that Sunday afternoon in 2008 and will never forget it. I was 20 years of age at the time and the weather was cold and drizzling. I was driving north when I lost control of my car and drove right through the middle of oncoming traffic. As my wheel locked up, I saw a big purple semi-tractor straight ahead coming full speed. I heard the horn of the big truck and it happened so fast that I couldn't pray. When we crashed the impact was if an elevator snapped its cords and dropped me to the ground. I could smell the burning rubber and my upper body got knocked over to the passenger side. I was dazed but I still was alert. I had blurred vision, trouble breathing, and was drifting in and out. I wasn't in pain but I cried for help. A few minutes later the firefighters arrived on my passenger window. They asked me a couple of questions before I passed out and took a long nap. It took 15 rescuers to cut me free from the wreckage. I broke everything from my neck down. When I woke up, I had a tube in my neck, a broken clavicle, a cracked sternum, eight broken ribs, a punctured lung, a broken elbow, a broken femur, and both ankles were shattered. I was hospitalized for two weeks and was transferred to a nursing facility where I spent four months learning how to walk again. Now I can walk and do almost everything I've done beforehand. I'm physically okay but suffer a lot of anxiety. See, I was in a no fault accident about ten years ago, which resulted in the death of the other driver. As a result of both these accidents, I developed fibromyalgia, chronic fatigue, severe insomnia, depression, anxiety, and other symptoms of PTSD. The more recent accident made me feel even worse and brought back a lot of vivid memories.

This recent accident recreated the memories I had been fighting to get rid of for ten years and I have nightmares and sleep issues. For a while, I had to stop physical therapy because of pain and received one injection after another. But I continued psychotherapy and have been working through the issues raised by both accidents. My psychotherapist has been having me lecture groups of young people about how to avoid accidents. For example, I did not wear a safety belt in either accident. You would think that I would have learned the first time, but I didn't. And when I had my first accident, I had been texting. But I did stop texting while driving and tell young people to do the same. I have not been able to work full-time since my second accident but spend a lot of time giving talks. The students I speak to are so upset when they hear my story, they promise to drive carefully, use a safety belt, avoid texting, and—of course—never drive while under the influence of any type of alcohol, illegal drug, or medication. I guess something positive has come out of my ordeal. I may even have saved some lives.

Saleh Bien's story is a dramatic one. But his popular series of lectures has created something positive out of what could have been an overwhelmingly negative experience.Post-traumatic strengths can reframe a trauma into a triumph, and can even reduce or erase the array of symptoms that accompany PTSD.

We will close our book on this optimistic note. Trauma is part of the human condition, but post-traumatic strengths are part of the human heritage. In the words of one of the Haitian artists who survived the 2010 earthquake and the destruction of some of his favorite paintings, "Let's get on with it. Tomorrow is another day."

# Timeline

| | |
|---|---|
| **1900 B.C.E.** | Trauma-induced psychological distress was reported by an Egyptian physician who wrote of "hysterical" reactions to trauma. |
| **480–490 B.C.E.** | Herodotus reported Greek soldiers' severe reactions to combat stress and shame as being "out of heart" to continue fighting in battles. |
| **1003** | The *Anglo-Saxon Chronicles* described an English commander who was unable to lead his troops because of nausea. |
| **1666** | Samuel Pepys wrote about the Great Fire of London and people's fear that put them "out of their wits." |
| **1678** | Swiss military physicians used the term "nostalgia" in referring to a constellation of behaviors that followed combat stress. At about the same time, German physicians began referring to the condition as "homesickness." |
| **1727** | During the siege of Gibraltar, a soldier kept a diary in which he described his comrades' states of "extreme physical |

fatigue" leading to irrational thinking and behavior, even suicide. About the same time, a French physician Larrey described the condition as having three stages: (1) heightened excitement and imagination, (2) fever and gastrointestinal symptoms, and finally (3) depression and frustration.

**1860s**     The terms "nostalgia," "soldier's heart," and "exhausted heart" were used by physicians to describe soldiers experiencing combat stress during the U.S. Civil War.

**1863**      The first military hospital for the "insane" was established by the Union military, the primary diagnosis being "nostalgia." The hospital was closed at the end of the war and "insane" veterans were released into the countryside, producing public outcry.

**1864**      The Assistant U.S. Surgeon General announced that most veterans who claimed to suffer symptoms of war trauma were malingering.

**1865**      Charles Dickens was involved in a railway accident, suffering symptoms of what today would be called posttraumatic stress; he attributed his long-lasting "unsteady" condition to the accident saying he was "not quite right within." Railway accident victims began suing railroads but the railroads attributed this to "compensation neurosis," the attempt to get something for nothing.

**1875**      A system of "soldier's homes" was set up around the country for veterans suffering from combat stress. Soon thereafter, the director of the Tongus, Maine "home" noted that the demand for services increased rather than decreased over time.

**1905**      The Russian Army's attempt to diagnose and treat "battle shock" following the war with Japan represents the birth of military psychiatry. Even after treatment, less than 20 percent were able to return to battle.

**1914–1919** The labels "shell shock," "neurasthenia," and "effort syndrome" were used to describe World War I soldiers' experience with war-related trauma. Freud used the term "war neurosis," attributing the problem to a conflict between a soldier's "war ego" and "peace ego." U.S. psychiatrists attributed the condition to men who were "weak in character."

1940s    The terms "combat stress reaction," "combat exhaustion," and "battle fatigue" were used to describe traumatic stress associated with World War II. Military screening rejected some five million recruits on the basis of psychiatric screening.

1950s    Of some 200,000 Americans seeing combat in the Korean Police Action, one in four became psychiatric casualties.

1952     The *Diagnostic and Statistical Manual of Mental Disorders (DSM)* is published by the American Psychiatric Association and "gross stress reaction" is recognized as an official diagnosis in relationship to traumatic stress during war for both war veterans and civilians.

1960s    Of the 2.8 million Americans serving in Vietnam, 480,000 developed full-blown stress reactions while another 350,000 had partial stress reactions.

1968     The *Diagnostic and Statistical Manual of Mental Disorders* (2nd edition; *DSM-II*) is published. "Gross stress reaction" is removed from the diagnostic manual in favor of "transient situational disturbances." The definition of "anxiety neurosis" is related not only to war and combat, but to sexual abuse, car accidents, natural disasters, genocide, etc.

1980     The *Diagnostic and Statistical Manual of Mental Disorders* (3rd edition; *DSM-III*) is published. "Post-traumatic stress disorder" is officially recognized in the diagnostic literature within the "anxiety disorder" nomenclature category

1989     The National Center for PTSD is created to promote the education and treatment of post-traumatic stress disorder.

2005     The National Comorbidity Survey reported that the lifetime prevalence of PTSD among adults in the United States is 6 to 8 percent.

2006     The American Psychological Association developed "The Road to Resilience," a set of materials to help families and communities deal with the threat of terrorism and reactions to it.

2007                A U.S. Department of Defense survey revealed that nine out of ten psychologists treating PTSD in the Veterans Administration system do not use exposure therapy or any of the other evidence-based treatments recommended by the U.S. government.

2010                The rate of suicide among veterans increases every year since records were first kept in 1974. The rate is especially high among veterans returning from Iraq and Afghanistan.

2010                Data from the National Comorbidity Survey revealed that at least four out of ten adults in the United States reported having experienced at least one potentially traumatizing event by the age of 13.

# Glossary

**Avoidance** is a common symptom of post-traumatic stress disorder (PTSD). When a person avoids, he or she attempts to keep away from, escape from, or shun elements associated with the traumatizing event. Some of these reminders can include similar locations, sounds, smells, and any other particular trigger connected to elements of the trauma.

**Comorbidity** is the simultaneous presence in an individual of two or more mental or physical disorders or illnesses. For example, an individual with a PTSD diagnosis might also be diagnosed with a traumatic brain injury and an obsessive-compulsive disorder.

**Coping styles** are strategic behaviors that people adopt to navigate their way through difficult situations. In the case of PTSD, adaptive coping styles would include engaging in athletic activity, the creative or performing arts, social activities, and spiritual or religious practices. Maladaptive coping styles would include alcohol or substance abuse, social isolation, engaging in unprotected and/or promiscuous sexual activity, and risky, life-threatening behaviors.

**Differential diagnosis** is the process of determining which of two or more disorders with overlapping symptoms characterize a person.

**The experiencer** is the person who is experiencing a potentially traumatizing event. The initiation of PTSD relies upon the experiencer's exposure to a potentially traumatizing event and his or her reaction to that exposure. At this point, the event becomes a traumatizing event, and the reaction becomes a traumatic experience. This reaction involves the direct experience of trauma (a motor vehicle accident, a natural disaster, sexual abuse, torture, war combat, etc.) another person's death, or the actual or threatened death or serious injury (physical or psychological) to the experiencer or a person being witnessed by the experiencer. This can include learning about an unexpected or violent death, serious harm, or threat of death or injury of another person, even someone not emotionally close to the experiencer (some writers refer to this as secondary or vicarious PTSD).

**Extinction** refers to the systematic removal of negative emotional reactions from an experience through such procedures as emotional processing or the discontinuation of reinforcement. If it does not occur naturally, it is an important goal of practitioners who treat PTSD.

**Fear memories** are specific recollections of the traumatizing event marked by intense fear, anxiety, and/or terror. This fear memory is extremely resistant to being integrated into the fabric of one's everyday life.

**The fight or flight response** (or fight–flight reaction) is defined by the *American Psychological Association Dictionary of Psychology* as an emotional and visceral response to an emergency that mobilizes energy for attacking or avoiding the offending stimulus. It is characterized by a pattern of physiological changes in the sympathetic nervous system in response to stress that leads to mobilization of energy for fighting or fleeing the situation.

**Post-traumatic stress disorder (PTSD)** is a term that first appeared in 1980 in the American Psychiatric Association's *Diagnostic and Statistical Manual of Mental Disorders* (DSM, 3rd and 4th editions, 1980 and 1994) and in 1977 in the World Health Organization's *International Statistical Classification of Diseases and Related Health Problems* (ICD, 9th and 10th editions, 1977 and 1992). While these classification systems are used throughout the world, they reflect Western cultural beliefs about human nature; thus, it is necessary to consider cultural implications when a mental health practitioner makes a formal diagnosis. In many non-Western societies, a traditional healer might use such terms as "soul loss" to refer to conditions that resemble PTSD among Westerners. For a diagnosis of PTSD to be applied, the experiencer's response to a traumatizing event entails intense anxiety, fear, helplessness, shame, or agitation. The latter is especially common among children with PTSD and impairs their ability to concentrate and pay attention. Responses to the trauma typically include frequent re-experiencing of the traumatic experience (as in nightmares and "flashbacks"), avoidance of reminders associated with the trauma, numbing or emotional responsiveness, and persistent symptoms of arousal. This latter condition is often referred to as hyperarousal, as in an increased heart rate or sleep disorders such as insomnia.

**The PTSD spectrum** ranges from traumatic stress reactions, which are both normal and temporary, to complex PTSD, which is long-lasting and severe, resulting from several forms of trauma or from repeated trauma. In subliminal PTSD, life stressors have triggered a number of symptoms but not enough to qualify for a PTSD diagnosis. Acute PTSD is marked by six or more symptoms but lasts for three months or less. Chronic PTSD is also characterized by six or more symptoms but lasts for more than three months, sometimes for a lifetime. Somewhat off the spectrum is delayed-onset PTSD, in which symptoms do not develop until after six months, and secondary PTSD. In addition to this longitudinal spectrum, there is a spectrum of severity, ranging from mild to severe. Two people, one with acute PTSD and one with chronic PTSD, may have six or more symptoms, but they may be severe in the former case and mild in the latter case. Typically, there are predisposing, activating, and maintaining aspects of PTSD. However, some individuals manifest severe symptomology even though their activating stressors are not generally thought to be traumatizing. And there are others who lack predisposing factors, such as abusive or otherwise unpleasant childhood experiences, whose condition was brought about solely by the traumatizing event. The term "peri-traumatic" is often used to describe those aspects of a traumatizing event that activated the PTSD.

**Recurrent nightmares** can be non-traumatic or traumatic. A non-traumatic nightmare is not evoked from a traumatic fear memory; rather, it is associated with negative and anxiety-producing experiences such as the fear of giving a speech or taking an examination. This anxiety brings about major stimulation of the body during sleep. Most people diagnosed with PTSD commonly experience traumatic nightmares. Traumatic nightmares cannot be processed through natural means of extinction and remain "stuck" as the brain tries, in vain, to extinguish them night after night. The defining point between the two types of nightmares is that non-traumatic nightmares *are* regulated through extinction.

**Re-experiencing** the traumatizing event is a key diagnostic symptom. It encompasses recurrent intrusive thoughts about the event, nightmares about the event, and spontaneous flashbacks in which the event is relived.

**Trauma** is a word that originated in the late 17th century and is derived from the Greek word for "wound." In the most general sense, a wound implies that an injury has occurred. Sometimes this injury may be physical, and at other times it may be psychological. Although psychological wounding—an injury to the psyche due to a traumatizing event— can occur along with a physical wound, bodily harm is not necessary for an emotional reaction to occur. The intensity (minor or major) of wounding that occurs is directly connected to how an individual experiences, thinks, and feels about a traumatizing encounter, activity, or occurrence. The American Psychological Association's *Dictionary of Psychology* defines trauma as an occurrence in which a person witnesses or experiences a threat to his or her own life or physical safety or to that of others and experiences fear, terror, or helplessness. Such occurrences challenge an individual's view of the world as a just, safe, and predictable place.

**A traumatizing event** is an incident or injury that challenges an individual's capacity to cope with or integrate the event. A **traumatic experience** is one that overwhelms the individual's capacity to cope with or integrate a traumatizing event, an experience that challenges one's existential worldview or the personal mythology that has helped the individual make sense of his or her life. The traumatizing event need not have been life-threatening; taunting, teasing, and bullying, for example, may be traumatic even though they do not necessarily lead to physical danger. They may however, evoke a traumatic experience that drastically disrupted one's view of the world as a friendly place in which one is welcome and secure. Traumatic experiences often result in shame and a loss of status among one's peers—an outcome that can be devastating to adolescents. We have differentiated traumatizing events and traumatic experiences. A catastrophic event such as a car crash is *potentially traumatizing* to the occupants of that car. Some people will assimilate the experience and bounce back easily. For others, that event will become *traumatizing* and will become a *traumatic experience*. An event usually is a shared incident, something that a group of people have in common. But each participant or onlooker may experience that event in a different way. What is stressful for one person may be run-of-the-mill for another. Therefore, we have used the term "traumatizing event" to describe what is extremely stressful for a particular person; we use the term "traumatic experience" to refer to a person's subjective reaction to that event.

**Triggers** are environmental cues that are similar to the original traumatizing event and can signal a recollection, causing significant impairment to one's functioning. Some triggers might be as subtle as recognizing a familiar smell, finding oneself in a crowded street or elevator, or even hearing a loud noise that resembles the traumatizing event or events.

# Bibliography

Abramowitz, J. S., Deacon, B. J., & Whiteside, S. H. (2011). *Exposure therapy for anxiety: Principles and practice*. New York: Guilford Press.

American Psychiatric Association. (1980). *Diagnostic and statistical manual of mental disorders (DSM-III)*. Washington, DC: American Psychiatric Association.

American Psychiatric Association. (2000). *Diagnostic and statistical manual of mental disorders, DSM-IV-TR* (4th ed., text revision). Washington, DC: American Psychiatric Association.

Arehart-Treichel, J. (2004). Brain activation may explain PTSD flashbacks. *Psychiatric News, 39*, p. 61.

Aristizabal, H., & Lefer, D. (2010). *The blessing next to the wound: A story of art, activism, and transformation*. Herndon, VA: Lantern Books.

Arons, S. (2003). Self-therapy through personal writing: A study of Holocaust victims' diaries and memoirs. In S. Krippner & T.M. McIntyre (Eds.), *The psychological impact of war trauma on civilians: An international perspective* (pp. 123–133). Westport, CT: Praeger.

Balaban, V. (2009). Assessment of children. In Foa, E.B., Keane, T.M., Friedman, M.J., & Cohen, J.A. (Eds.), *Effective treatments for PTSD* (pp. 62–80). New York: Guilford Press.

Barrett, D., & Behbehani, J. (2003). Post-traumatic nightmares in Kuwait following the Iraqi invasion. In S. Krippner & T.M. McIntyre (Eds.), *The psychological impact of war trauma on civilians* (pp. 135–141). Westport, CT: Praeger.

Bartholomew, K., & Horowitz, L. (1991). Attachment styles among young adults: A test of a four-category model. *Journal of Personality and Social Psychology, 61*, 226–244.

Baum, D. (2004). The price of valor. *The New Yorker*, pp. 44–52.

Bazar, J. (1991, October). Abused children show signs of PTSD. *Monitor on Psychology*, p. 3.

Beck, A.T. (1976). *Cognitive therapy and the emotional disorders*. New York: International Universities Press.

Beck, A.T., & Emery, G. (1985). *Anxiety disorder and phobias: A cognitive perspective*. New York: Basic Books.

Beck, J.S. (2011). *Cognitive behavior therapy: Basics and beyond* (2nd ed.). New York: Guilford.

Belasco, A. (2007). *The cost of Iraq, Afghanistan, and other global war on terror operations since 9/11*. Washington, DC: Congressional Research Service.

Benish, S., Imel, Z., & Wampold, B. (2008). The relative efficacy of bona fide psychotherapies for treating post-traumatic stress disorder: A meta-analysis of direct comparisons. *Clinical Psychology Review, 28*, 746–758.

Berkowitz, S.J., Stover, C.S., & Marans, S.R. (2011). The Child and Family Traumatic Stress Intervention: Secondary prevention for youth at risk of developing PTSD. *Journal of Child Psychology and Psychiatry, 52*, 676–685.

Bowlby, J. (1988). *A secure base: Parent-child attachment and healthy human development*. New York: Basic Books.

Bremner, J.D., & Marmar, C. (Eds.). (1998). *Trauma, memory, and dissociation*. Washington, DC: American Psychiatric Association Press.

Briere, J. (2004). *Psychological assessment of adult post-traumatic states: Phenomenology, diagnosis, and measurement* (2nd ed.). Washington, DC: American Psychological Association.

Brinkley, J. (2011). *Cambodia's curse: The modern history of a troubled land*. New York: Public Affairs Books.

Brown, D., Scheflin, A.W., & Hammond, D. C. (1998). *Memory, trauma treatment, and the law*. New York: W.W. Norton.

Brown, L.S. (2008). *Cultural competence in trauma therapy: Beyond the flashback*. Washington, DC: American Psychological Association.

Brubaker, B. (2010, September). The art of resilience. *The Smithsonian*, pp. 37–45.

Budden, A. (2009). The role of shame in post-traumatic stress disorder: A proposal for a socio-emotional model for DSM-V. *Social Science and Medicine, 69*, 1032–1039.

Burkett, B.G., & Whitley, G. (1998). *Stolen valor: How the Vietnam generation was robbed of its heroes and its history*. Dallas, TX: Verity.

Cahill, S. P., Rothbaum, B. O., Resick, P. A., & Follette, V. M. (2009). Cognitive behavioral therapy for adults. In E. B. Foa, T. M. Keane, M. J. Friedman, & J. A. Cohen (Eds.), *Effective treatments for PTSD* (pp. 139–222). New York: The Guilford Press.

Carlat, D.J. (2010). *Psychiatry as Faust: Has psychiatry sold its soul to the pharmaceutical industry?* New York: Free Press.

Carlson, E.B., & Rosser-Hogan, R. (1991). Trauma experiences, post-traumatic stress, dissociation, and depression in Cambodian refugees. *American Journal of Psychiatry, 148*, 1548–1551.

Carrion, V.G., Weems, C.F., Ray, R., & Reiss, A.L. (2002). Toward an empirical definition of pediatric PTSD: The phenomenology of PTSD symptoms in youth. *Journal of the American Academy of Child and Adolescent Psychiatry, 41*, 166–173.

Chamberlin, J. (2010, October). "I swore I'd never tell." *Monitor on Psychology*, 54–55.

Clancy, S. (2010). *The trauma myth: The truth about sexual abuse of children*. New York: Basic Books.

Davies, J.A. (2011). *Relational dharma: A liberating path of higher human relatedness and freedom*. Vancouver, Canada: Scholarly Research Press.

Dean, E.T., Jr. (1997). *Shook over Hell: Post-traumatic stress, Vietnam, and the Civil War*. Cambridge, MA: Harvard University Press.

Deykin, E.Y. (1999). Posttraumatic Stress Disorder in Childhood and Adolescence: A Review. *MedGenMed 1*(3), [formerly published in Medscape Psychiatry & Mental Health eJournal 4(3), 1999]. Available at: http://www.medscape.com/viewarticle/430606

Donnelly, C. L. (2009). Psychopharmacology for children and adolescents. In E. B. Foa, T. M. Keane, M. J. Friedman, & J. A. Cohen (Eds.), *Effective treatments for PTSD* (pp. 269–278). New York: Guilford Press.

Ehlers, A., Bisson, J., Clark, D.M., Creaner, M., Pilling, S., Richards, D., Schnurr, P.P., Turner, S., & Yule, W. (2010). Do all psychological treatments really work the same in post-traumatic stress disorder? *Clinical Psychology Review, 30*, 269–276.

Eisenhart, R.W. (1977). Flower of the dragon: An example of applied humanistic psychology. *Journal of Humanistic Psychology, 17*, 3–24.

Elliot, R., & Greenberg, L.S. (2001). Process-experiential psychotherapy. In D.J. Cain (Ed.), *Humanistic psychotherapies: Handbook of research and practice* (pp. 279–306). Washington, DC: American Psychological Association.

Ellis, A. (1957). Outcome of employing three techniques of psychotherapy. *Journal of Clinical Psychology, 13*(4), 344–350.

Ellis, A., & Ellis, D.J. (2011). *Rational emotive behavior therapy*. Washington, DC: APA Books.

Feder, A., Southwick, S.M., Goetz, R.R., Wang, Y., Alonso, A., Smith, B.W., & Vythilingam, M. (2008). Post-traumatic growth in former Vietnam prisoners of war. *Psychiatry, 71*, 359–370. doi:10.1521/psyc.2008.71.4.359

Feinstein, D., & Krippner, S. (2008). *Personal mythology* (3rd ed.). Santa Rosa, CA: Energy Psychology Press.

Finnegan, W. (2008). The last tour. *The New Yorker*, 64–71.

Foa, E.B., Gilboa-Schechtman, E., & Rothbaum, B.O. (2007). *Prolonged exposure therapy for PTSD: Emotional processing of traumatic experiences therapist guide*. New York: Oxford University Press.

Fretwell, P., & Baldwin-Kiland, T. (2011). History is on Japan's side. *The New York Times*. Retrieved from http://www.nytimes.com/2011/03/16/opinion/16iht edfretwell16.html

Friedman, M.J., Davidson, H.R.T., & Stein, D.J. (2009). Psychopharmacotherapy for adults. In E.B. Foa, T.M. Keane, M.J. Friedman, & J.A. Cohen (Eds.), *Effective treatments for PTSD* (pp. 245–268). New York: Guilford.

Fuchsman, K. (2008). Traumatized soldiers. *Journal of Psychohistory, 36*, 73–84.

Gelso, C. J. (2011). *The real relationship in psychotherapy*. Washington, DC: APA Books.

Gilbertson, M.W., Shenton, M.E., Ciszewski, A., Kasai, K., Lasko, N.B. Orr, S.P., & Pitman, R.K. (2002). Smaller hippocampal volume predicts pathologic vulnerability to psychological trauma. *Nature Neuroscience*, 1242–1247.

Goldstein, A. (2001, October 15). Even soldiers hurt. *TIME*, 84.

Grof, S. (1985). *Beyond the brain: Birth, death, and transcendence in psychotherapy*. Albany, NY: State University of New York Press.

Greening, T. (1997). Post-traumatic stress disorder: An existential humanistic perspective. In S. Krippner & S.M. Powers, (Eds.), *Broken images, broken selves: Dissociative narratives in clinical practice* (pp. 125–135). New York: Brunner/Mazel.

Greer, M. (2005, April). A new kind of war. *Monitor on Psychology*, 38–40.

Hamblen, J., & Barnet, E. (2009). *PTSD in children and adolescents.* National Center for PTSD. http://www.ptsd.va.gov/professional/pages/ptsd_in_children_and _adolescents_overview_for_professionals.asp

Han, J.H., Kushner, S.A., Yiu, A.P., Hsiang, H.L., Buch, T., Waisman, A., Bontempi, B., Neve, R.L., Frankland, P.W., & Josselyn, S.A. (2009). Selective erasure of a fear memory, *Science, 323*, 1492–1495.

Hartmann, E. (1984). *The nightmare: The psychology and the biology of terrifying dreams.* New York: Basic Books.

Hayward, P. (2008). Traumatic brain injury: The signature of modern conflicts. *Lancet Neurology, 7*, 200–201.

Herman, J. (1997). *Trauma and recovery* (2nd ed.). New York: Basic Books.

Herman, J.L., & Schatzow, E. (1987). Recovery and verification of memories of childhood sexual trauma. *Psychoanalytic Psychology, 4*, 1–14.

Hoge, C.W., Castro, C.A., Messer, S.C., McGurk, D., Cotting, D.I., & Koffman, R.L. (2004). Combat duty in Iraq and Afghanistan, mental health problems, and barriers to care. *New England Journal of Medicine, 351*, 13–22.

Ireland, R.R. (2005). *Suicide prevention and suicide rates.* Washington, DC: Office of Assistant Secretary of Defense.

Janoff-Bulman, R. (1992). *Shattered assumptions: Towards a new psychology of trauma.* New York: Free Press.

Kanas, N. (2005). Group therapy for patients with chronic traumatic related stress disorders. *International Journal of Group Psychotherapy, 55*, 161–166.

Kaplan, A. (2006). Hidden combat wounds: Extensive, deadly, costly. *Psychiatric Times, 25*, 1–3.

Kardiner, A. (1941). *The traumatic neuroses of war.* New York: Hoeber.

Keane, T.M., Kolb, L.C., Kaloupek, D.G., Orr, S.P., Blanchard, E.B. et al. (1998). Utility of psychophysiological measurement in the diagnosis of post-traumatic stress disorder: Results from a Department of Veterans Affairs Cooperative Study. *Journal of Consulting Psychology, 66*, 914–923.

Kessler, R.C., Sonnega, A., Bromet, E., Hughes, M., & Nelson, C.B. (1995). Post-traumatic stress disorder in the National Comorbidity Survey. *Archives of General Psychiatry, 52*, 1048–1060.

Krippner, S., & McIntyre, T.M. (Eds.). (2003). *The psychological impact of war trauma on civilians.* Westport, CT: Praeger.

Krippner, S., & Paulson, D. S. (2006). Post-traumatic stress disorder among U.S. combat veterans. In T. G. Plante (Ed.), *Mental disorders of the new millennium: Public and social problems* (Vol. 2, pp. 1–23). Westport, CT: Praeger.

Krystal, J. H., Rosenheck, R. A., Cramer, J. A., Vessicchio, J. C., Jones, K. M., Vertrees, J. E., Horney, R. A., Huang, G. D., Stock, C. (2011). 15. Adjunctive risperidone treatment for antidepressant-resistant symptoms of chronic military service-related PTSD: a randomized trial. *The Journal of the American Medical Association, 306*, 493–502.

Kudler, H.S., Krupnick, J.L., Blank, A.S. Jr., Herman, J.L., & Horowitz, M.J. (2009). Psychodynamic therapy for adults. In E.B. Foa, T.M. Keane, M.J. Friedman, & J.A. Cohen (Eds.), *Effective treatments for PTSD* (pp. 349–369). New York: Guilford.

Kulka, R.A., Schlenger, W.E., Fairbank, J.A., Hough, R.L., Jordan. B.K., Marmar, C.R., & Weiss, D.S. (1990). *Trauma and the Vietnam War generation: Report of the findings from the National Vietnam Veterans Readjustment Study.* New York: Brunner/Mazel.

Laing, R.D. (1965). *The divided self: An existential study in sanity and madness.* New York: Pelican Books.

Laing, R.D. (1983). *The politics of experience.* New York: Pantheon.

Lanius, R. A., Williamson, P. C., Densmore, M., Boksman, K., Neufeld, R. W., Gati, J. S., & Menon, R. S. (2004). The Nature of Traumatic Memories: A 4-T fMRI Functional Connectivity Analysis. *American Journal of Psychiatry. 161*(1), 36–44.

Lapin, D. (1997). Dissociation in terror of death: The "hypnoid state" revisited. In S. Krippner & S.M. Powers (Eds.), *Broken images, broken selves: Dissociative narratives in clinical practice* (pp. 248–273). Washington, DC: Brunner Mazel.

Leeies, M., Pagura, J., Sareen, J., & Bolton, J.M. (2010). The use of alcohol and drugs to self-medicate symptoms of post-traumatic stress disorder. *Depression and Anxiety, 27,* 731–736.

Leopold, J. (2011, January 5). Army's "Spiritual Fitness" Test comes under fire [Online news site]. Retrieved from http://www.truth-out.org/armys-fitness-test designed -psychologist-who-inspired-cias-torture-program-under fire66577

Levin, R., & Nielson, T.A. (2007). Disturbed dreaming post-traumatic stress disorder, and affect distress: A review and neurocognitive model. *Psychological Bulletin, 133,* 482–528.

Lieberman, A.F., & Van Horn, P. (2008). *Psychotherapy with infants and young children: Repairing the effects of stress and trauma on early attachment.* New York: Guildford Press.

Lindley, S.E., Carlson, E.B., & Benoit, M. (2004). Basal and dexamethasone suppressed salivary cortisol concentrations in a community sample of patients with posttraumatic stress disorder. *Biological Psychiatry 55*(9), 940–945.

Lopez, F., Melendez, M., Sauer, E., Berger, E., & Wyssmann, J. (1998). Internal working models, self-reported problems, and help-seeking attitudes among college students. *Journal of Counseling Psychology, 45,* 79–83.

Luborsky, L.B., Crits-Christophe, P., Mintz, J., and Auerbach, A. (1988). *Who will benefit from psychotherapy?* New York: Basic Books.

Macklin, M.L., Metzher, L.G., Litz, B.T., McNally, R.J., Lasko, N.B. et al. (1998). Lower pre-combat intelligence is a risk factor for post-traumatic stress disorder. *Journal of Consulting and Clinical Psychology, 66,* 323–326.

MacLean, A. (2010). The things they carry: Combat, disability, and unemployment among US men. *American Sociological Review, 75*(4), 563–585.

Marciniak, R.D. (1986). Implications to forensic psychiatry of post-traumatic stress disorder: A review. *Military Medicine, 151,* 434–437.

Marlowe, D.H. (2001). *Psychological and psychosocial consequences of combat and deployment, with special emphasis on the Gulf War.* Washington, DC: The RAND Corporation.

McCann, I.I., & Pearlman, L.A. (1990). *Psychological trauma and the adult survivor: Theory, therapy, and transformation.* New York: Brunner-Mazel.

McKinney, K. (2007). Breaking the conspiracy of silence: Testimony, traumatic memory, and psychotherapy with survivors of political violence. *Ethos, 35,* 265–279.

McNally, R.J. (2003). Progress and controversy in the study of post-traumatic stress disorder. *American Review of Psychology, 54,* 229–252.

Mehl-Madrona, L. (2010). *Healing the mind through the power of story: The promise of narrative psychiatry.* Rochester, NY: Bear.

Mendelson, G. (1987). The concept of post-traumatic stress disorder: A review. *International Journal of Law and Psychiatry, 10*, 45–62.

Milliken, C.S., Auchterlonie, J.L., & Hoge, C.W. (2007). Longitudinal assessment of mental health problems among Active and Reserve Component soldiers returning from the Iraq War. *Journal of the American Medical Association, 298*, 2141–2148.

Orr, S.P., Pitnam, R.R., Gilbertson, M.W., Shenton, M.E., Cisewski, A., Kasai, K., & Lasko, N.B. (2002). Smaller hippocampal volume predicts pathologic vulnerability to psychological trauma. *Nature Neuroscience, 5*, 1742–1747.

Osofsky, J.D., & Lieberman, A.F. (2011). A call for integrating a mental health perspective into systems of care for abused and neglected infants and young children. *American Psychologist, 86*, 120–158.

Ozer, E.J., & Weiss, D.S. (2004). Who develops post-traumatic stress disorder? *Current Directions in Psychological Science, 13*, 169–172.

Paulson, D.S. (1994). *Walking the point: Myth, male initiation, and the Vietnam veteran.* Plantation, FL: Distinctive Publishing.

Paulson, D.S., & Krippner, S. (2007). *Haunted by combat: Understanding PTSD in war veterans.* Westport, CT: Praeger Security International.

Paulson, D.S., & Krippner, S. (2009). *Haunted by combat: Understanding PTSD in war veterans* (updated edition). Lanham, MD: Rowman & Littlefield.

Payne, J.D., & Kensinger, E.A. (2010). Sleep's role in the consolidation of emotional episodic memories. *Current Directions in Psychological Science, 19*, 290–295.

Peterson, A.L., Luethcke, C.A., Borah, E.V., Borah, A.M., Young-McCaughan, S. (2011) Assessment and treatment of combat-related PTSD in returning war veterans. *The Journal of Clinical Psychology in Medical Settings. 18*(2), 164–175.

Pitchford, D.B. (2009). *An existential study of Iraq War veterans' traumatizing experiences* (Doctoral dissertation). Available from Proquest Dissertations and Theses database. (UMI No. 3339401)

Pitchford, D.B. (2009). The neuropsychology of nightmares reported by Iraq War veterans. In S. Krippner & D.J. Ellis (Eds.), *Perchance to dream: Frontiers of dream psychology* (pp. 113–132). Hauppauge, NY: Nova Science.

Pitchford, D.B. (2009a). The existentialism of Rollo May: An influence on trauma treatment. *Journal of Humanistic Psychology, 49*(4), 441–461.

Pizarro, J., Silver, R.C., & Prause, J. (2006). Physical and mental health costs of traumatic war experiences among Civil War veterans. *Archives of General Psychiatry, 63*, 193–200.

Rank, O. (1929). *The trauma of birth.* New York: Harcourt Brace.

Rosen, G.M. (1995). The Aleutian Enterprise sinking and post-traumatic stress disorder: Misdiagnosis in clinical and forensic settings. *Professional Psychology: Research and Practice, 26*, 82–87.

Rosenheck, R., & Fontana, A. (1999). Changing patterns of care for war-related post-traumatic stress disorder at Department of Veterans Affairs Medical Centers: The use of performance data to guide program development. *Military Medicine, 164*, 795–802.

Saigh, P.A., & Bremner, D. (Eds.). (1999). *Post-traumatic stress disorder: A comprehensive text.* Needham Heights, MA: Allyn & Bacon.

Salter, E., & Stallard, P. (2011). The psychological impact of traumatic events on children. *Psychological Injury & Law, 1*, 138–146.

Sapolsky, R.M. (1996). Why stress is bad for your brain. *Science, 273,* 749–750.

Savage, D., & Miller, T. (2011). *It gets better.* New York: Dutton.

Schmahl, C., Berne, K., Krause, A., Kleindienst, N., Valerius, G., Vermetten, E., & Bohus, M. (2009). Hippocampus and amygdala volumes in patients with borderline personality disorder with or without post-traumatic stress disorder. *Journal of Psychiatry and Neuroscience, 34(4),* 289–295.

Schultz, J.M., Tallman, B.A., & Altmaier, E.M. (2010). Pathways to posttraumatic growth: The contributions of forgiveness and importance of religion and spirituality. *Psychology of Religion and Spirituality, 2,* 104–114.

Schuster, M.A., Stein, B.D., Jaycox, L.H., Collins, R.L., Marshall, G.N., et al. (2001). A national survey of stress reactions after the September 11, 2001, terrorist attacks. *New England Journal of Medicine, 345,* 1507–1512.

Seligman, M.E.P., & Csikszentmihalyi, M. (2000). Positive psychology: An introduction. *American Psychologist, 55,* 5–14.

Selye, H. (1974). *Stress and distress.* Philadelphia, PA: J.B. Lippincott.

Shalev, A.Y., Sahar, T., Freedman, S., et al. (1998). A prospective study of heart rate responses following trauma and the subsequent development of post-traumatic stress disorder. *Archives of General Psychiatry, 55,* 553–559.

Silva, R.R., Alpert, M., Munoz, D.M., Singh, S., Matzner, F., & Dummitt, S. (2000). Stress and vulnerability to post-traumatic stress disorder in children and adolescents. *American Journal of Psychiatry, 157,* 1229–1235.

Smiley, L. (2010, November 3–9). Wounded pride. *San Francisco Weekly,* pp. 13–14, 17–18.

Solomon, S.D., & Johnson, D.M. (2002). Psychosocial treatment of post-traumatic stress disorder: A practice-friendly review of outcome research. *Journal of Clinical Psychology, 58,* 947–959.

Solomon, S., Greenberg, J., & Pyszczynski, T. (2003). Why war? Fear is the mother of violence. In S. Krippner & T.M. McIntyre (Eds.), *The psychological impact of war trauma on civilians: An international perspective* (pp. 299–309). Westport, CT: Praeger.

Southwick, S.M., Morgan, C.A. III, Nicholas, A.L., & Charney, D.S. (1997). Consistency of memory for combat-related traumatic events in veterans of Operation Desert Storm. *American Journal of Psychiatry, 154,* 173–177.

Spiegel, D. (1984). Multiple personality as a post-traumatic stress disorder. *Psychiatric Clinics of North America, 7,* 101–110.

Stallard P. (2006). Psychological interventions for post-traumatic reactions in children and young people: A review of randomised controlled trials. *Clinical Psychology Review, 26,* 895–911.

Stone, A. (1994, November 11). Some WWII vets fight enemy within. *USA Today,* 6A.

Tanielian, T., & Jaycox, L.H. (Eds.). (2008). *Invisible wounds of war: Psychological and cognitive injuries, their consequences, and the services to assist recovery.* Santa Monica, CA: RAND Corporation.

Tedeschi, R.G., & Calhoun, L.G. (1996). The Post-traumatic Growth Inventory: Measuring the positive legacy of trauma. *Journal of Traumatic Stress, 9,* 455–471.

Tedeschi, R.G., & McNally, J. (2011). Can we facilitate post-traumatic growth in combat veterans? *American Psychologist, 66(1),* 19–24.

Thabet, A.A.M., & Vostranis, P. (2005). Post traumatic stress disorder reactions in children or war: A longitudinal study. *Child Abuse and Neglect, 29,* 291–298.

van der Kolk, B.A. (1987). *Psychological trauma.* Washington, DC: American Psychiatric Press.

VandenBos, G.R. (Ed.). (2006). *APA dictionary of psychology.* Washington, DC: American Psychological Association.

Vasterling, J., & Brewin, C. (Eds.). (2005). *Neuropsychology of PTSD: Biological, cognitive, and clinical perspectives.* New York: Guilford Press.

Verrier, N. (1993). *The primal wound: Understanding the adopted child.* Baltimore, MD: Gateway Press.

Vitetta, L., Anton, B., Cortizo, F., & Sali, A. (2005). Mind-body medicine: Stress and its impact on overall health and longevity. *Annals of the New York Academy of Science, 1057,* 492–505.

Wasdin, H.E., & Templin, S. (2011). *SEAL team six: Memoirs of an elite Navy SEAL sniper.* New York: St. Martin's Press.

Weiderhold, B.K., & Weiderhold, M.D. (2004). *Virtual reality therapy for anxiety disorders: Advances in education and treatment.* Washington, DC: American Psychological Association Press.

White, N.P. (Ed.). (1983). *Handbook of Epictetus.* Indianapolis, IN: Hackett.

Williams, W.L. (1992). *The spirit and the flesh.* Boston, MA: Beacon Press.

World Health Organization. (1992). *International classification of diseases and related health problems,* 10th revision (ICD-10). Geneva, Switzerland: World Health Organization.

Yehuda, R., Teicher, M.H., Seckl, J.R., Grossman, R.A., Morris, A., & Bierer, L.M. (2007). Parental posttraumatic stress disorder as a vulnerability factor for low cortisol trait in offspring of holocaust survivors. *Archives of General Psychiatry, 64,* 1040–1048

Young, W.C. (1987). Emergence of a multiple personality in a post-traumatic stress disorder of adulthood. *American Journal of Clinical Hypnosis, 29,* 249–254.

Zimering, R., Munroe, J., & Gulliver, S.B. (2003). Secondary traumatization in mental health care providers. *Psychiatric Times, 20* (4), 43–47.

# Index

# About the Authors

**STANLEY KRIPPNER**, PhD, is the Alan Watts Professor of Psychology at Saybrook University in San Francisco, California. He is the recipient of the American Psychological Association's Award for Distinguished Contributions to the International Advancement of Psychology, the International Association for the Study of Dreams' Lifetime Achievement Award, and the Ashley Montagu Peace Award. His two dozen books include *Haunted by Combat: Understanding PTSD in War Veterans* and *The Psychological Impact of War on Civilians: An International Perspective*.

**DANIEL B. PITCHFORD**, PhD, is faculty at Saybrook University in San Francisco, CA. He supervises and teaches within the traumatic stress specialization / track for the PsyD program as well as for the university's College of Mind-Body Medicine and the College of Humanistic and Transpersonal Psychology. Dr. Pitchford also maintains a private practice providing individual counseling and consultation services on trauma as well as provides clinical supervision and management to Cascadia Behavioral Healthcare's enhanced care and outreach service programs for individuals struggling with severe mental and medical difficulties within the Springfield and Eugene, Oregon, areas. He has written and lectured on the fundamentals of suicide, PTSD, and traumatic stress, and also received the Rollo May Scholarship Award for his humanistic work with traumatic stress.

**JEANNINE DAVIES**, PhD, is a licensed psychotherapist and researcher based in Vancouver, B.C., Canada. She has taught and written on the areas of consciousness, human rights, and personal and social transformation. She is the founder of Relational Dharma, an intersubjective and integral model of consciousness, which is being applied as a means toward resolving individual and collective experiences of traumatic stress.